THE WORLD AT MY BACK
THOMAS MELLE

Translated from the German by LUISE VON FLOTOW

BIBLIOASIS
Windsor, Ontario

FIRST EDITION
10 9 8 7 6 5 4 3 2 1

Library and Archives Canada Cataloguing in Publication
Title: The world at my back / Thomas Melle ; translated from the German by
    Luise von Flotow.
Other titles: Welt im Rücken. English
Names: Melle, Thomas, 1975- author. | von Flotow, Luise, 1951- translator.
Series: Biblioasis international translation series ; no. 40.
Description: Series statement: Biblioasis international translation series ; no. 40
    Translation of: Die Welt im Rücken.
Identifiers: Canadiana (print) 20220474192 | Canadiana (ebook) 20220474249
    ISBN 9781771964517 (softcover) | ISBN 9781771964524 (EPUB)
Subjects: LCSH: Melle, Thomas, 1975- | LCSH: Authors, German—21st century—
    Biography. | LCSH: People with bipolar disorder—Germany—Biography.
    LCGFT: Autobiographies.
Classification: LCC PT2713.E48 Z46 2023 | DDC 838/.9203—dc23

Edited by Stephen Henighan and Daniel Wells
Copyedited by Chandra Wohleber
Typeset by Vanessa Stauffer
Cover designed by Natalie Olsen

The translation of this work was supported by a grant from the Goethe-Institut
in the framework of the "Books First" program.

PRINTED AND BOUND IN CANADA

PROLOGUE

I would like to tell you about a loss. My book collection. It no longer exists. I lost it.

The topic came up during a dinner held in my honour to celebrate a minor success. I was uncomfortable attending this dinner, but I didn't want to spoil the pleasure the organizers felt they were providing me. All in all, it turned out to be a successful event.

Henry, who in real life has a much lovelier name, was sitting next to me. I'd had a crush on her for a long time. We were talking like two people who trust each other, but I had the feeling that this was as much due to her gentle, calm manner as it was to any real intimacy. We were talking about literature, as we often had before, and instead of putting on my best, somewhat false front, I admitted I no longer owned a book collection.

The admission was an impulse I simply gave in to: for some time I had been more open about my losses and failures, even though these confessions were always accompanied by shame and stress. There is something vulgar about exhibiting your own catastrophes, but it's positively twisted to not acknowledge them when you're already reaping the consequences. Bertram, the host, caught this comment of mine from across the table and we talked about the slow, steady increase in the size of a book collection over the course of a life, and about the accumulation of stuff that, over the years, becomes an important part of some people's identity. We agreed that such a loss must be quite unbearable. Then the conversation fizzled out, and I turned back to Henry, to whom I still owed an explanation as to how my book collection had disappeared if I didn't want to leave a sizable gap in our conversation. And so, in a quieter tone than I'd usually use—although she also speaks quietly and was hard to understand, sitting as she was at my left, the side affected by tinnitus—I casually told her that I was bipolar. I expect she knew that already. Or she knew *something*. Everybody knew something.

The expression "elephant in the room" refers to a problem that is obvious and that is ignored. There's an elephant in the room that you can't overlook, but nobody talks about it. Maybe the elephant is embarrassing, maybe it's too present, maybe people think the elephant will go away again even though it's virtually squashing them up against the walls. My illness is such an elephant. The china (to let the elephant stomp through a second image) he has trampled is still tinkling under the soles of our shoes. But why talk of china? I'm the one who's been trampled.

I was once a collector. Addicted to culture, I had built up an impressive book collection that I kept updating and expanding over the decades, with a great eye for detail. My heart was in those books. I loved to feel all the writers who had influenced and inspired me at my back, and to have my contemporaries there too, with their new publications, letting me feel time move on and things change. I hadn't read all the books, but I needed them all, and I could check references or just get lost in one for the first time or all over again. My music collection had been just as impressive:

indie, electro, classical. These collections were part of my personality. It's strange how you can project yourself into the things around you. It's stranger still to toss them out without really wanting to.

In 2006 I sold the largest part of my collection, starting with the classical writers. Suddenly these much-loved books had become ballast the manic in me urgently needed to dump. In 2007, during my depression, I mourned this loss terribly. A collector had scattered the objects he was passionate about to the four winds and there was no getting them back. For three years I huddled amid my decimated collection, and then I went manic again. That was in 2010, and I sold off most of what was left of my truncated hoard along with all the CDs and records the dealers would take. I threw out the rest and got rid of a large pile of clothing as well. In 2011, I awoke from my delirium, emerged from the madness, and was dismayed at having lost and sold off everything I'd loved.

I still miss those books today. Usually I tell myself that even with a normal psychological constitution it would not have been all bad to trim down a book collection (but just trim it!) or that at some point I would have had enough of the constant archiving and hoarding and adopted a new, liberating minimalism: white walls, a sofa, a table with a Gerhard Richter–style candle on it, nothing more. But the decisions I made were due to illness. Not free will. And the empty walls, the echo in my apartment, still mock me today, and illustrate, to put it in plain terms, the destruction of an attempt at life.

Henry didn't know what to say. She looked at me, nodding, and then assured me that she was familiar with conditions such as mine, although she wouldn't dream of even beginning to compare my situation with hers. We talked some more about my condition and similar ones, the extreme highs and lows, without me wanting or being able to describe what my illness actually meant for my life. No further terrible details crossed my lips. The mention of my book collection would have to do for now. Still, it wasn't embarrassing to talk to her: there was obvious trust, as well as the start of a certain distancing. The illness, now it had a name, had clearly come between us, and yet I didn't regret having told her. Three or four weeks later we fell in love. But it didn't work out. She was scared of my illness, and I was afraid of her aristocratic family, almost narrow-minded in spite of its cosmopolitan allure, and so, after a week spent living in a dream, we knew there was no room for us in real life, though we carried on doggedly for a few more months, despite our own and other people's objections. Since then, I have only told her a few details of my story, though she is one of the people to whom I could and should tell everything. This book is dedicated to such impossibilities—and to a love that slipped away.

2

When I had sex with Madonna, I felt good for a moment. Madonna was still amazingly fit, but that didn't surprise me. We'd followed her transformation into a fitness machine around 2006 and seen her labour away in the "Hung Up" video, doing splits and squats, harder and harder, more and more extreme, a rubber person with softly contoured curves who wilfully shaped her body, thereby giving the spectre of physical decline a kick in its droopy ass. And now I was reaping the benefits of her exertions; I was being rewarded with the fruits of her sweat-inducing bodywork— while I had also lost a lot of weight over the past months and documented the process in detail on a blog I destroyed and rewrote every day. So things were all set, and I could just go pick her up in the Oranienstrasse. And why ever not? She'd been singing about me her whole life.

Björk too. But she'd really been getting on my nerves lately. She'd hang around me in bars and cafés, trying to touch my heart with her fractured, elfish singing. Hadn't she always been my true pop love? So why Madonna all of a sudden? That's what seemed to come whimpering out of her. In contrast to Madonna, Björk hadn't worked on herself as much, hadn't kept reinventing herself or sloughing off old skin. Björk seemed to think her Selma glasses from *Dancer in the Dark* along with her sloppy, worn-out, pathetic look could reignite my teenage love for her. She would approach me in dim cafés with leaves in her hair, coo something I couldn't understand, and disappear, mission unaccomplished. Likewise Courtney.

I can hardly remember the actual sex with Madonna. It was probably not particularly wild or particularly boring. Madonna is not a sex bomb, just as Elvis wasn't—one of his lovers once said that in bed he was like a baby, complete with the impulse to latch on to the motherly nipple. Madonna was also on an incestuous track and seemed to see me as her son, the fallen Jesus she wanted to perform oral sex on: *I'm on my knees / I'm gonna take you there,* and so our sex gave off an odour of the forbidden, without this heresy giving me the slightest kick. And soon I recognized the old woman under me, the flesh that was indeed softer, droopier to the touch, all masks gone, the crow's feet and laugh lines drawn deep into the skin. All masks gone, yes, except for the wolfish grin that had hit my reflection in the window of the bookstore. Madonna baring her long teeth. We'd been studying the books on display, our eyes had met, recognition on my part, a grin on hers, no further sign, and we were hurrying to my rundown apartment at the Kottbusser Tor, the wet asphalt like a dark mirror under our feet. She just came along. I remember how surprised I was that she was in good shape, almost like in the nude photos of the early eighties, but I have to admit that her breasts were much less prominent than expected, than the way the media or she herself had deliberately presented them. You had to subtract at least two cup sizes to get it right. But who was I to make such petty judgments, even as Madonna was literally disintegrating under my gaze? Or rather, who was I to disappoint her? We'd both spent decades waiting for this moment. So I skipped all further thoughts and evaluations and gave her what she took. The next morning she was gone, as her status required, without leaving a phone number. That's Madonna. I hadn't expected anything else.

I already knew about the way celebrities would come sneaking out of their hiding places. It was the same thing every time. I'd only just become aware of the unspeakable role I was playing. I'd only just begin to send out the right signals, and there they'd be, buzzing around me like stars around a black hole. And I devoured them all. Before I went for Madonna, MCA, the good, now unfortunately dead, MC of the Beastie Boys, had been slinking around to see what I was up to that damned godforsaken night. In contrast to Werner Herzog, who was always stalking me, MCA was pure, the soul of integrity. A brief thumbs-up let me know everything was okay, and so Madonna and I were able to go at it with a clear conscience. Because MCA was the personified conscience of pop, and what he approved of was politically and morally correct, no matter what the drag queens at the Roses bar might hiss in our direction, or what the young Turks at Oregano might say as they kept a baleful eye on the queens, dissing them with predictable slurs.

Let them figure out their contemptuous act on their own; it had nothing to do with us. Although, who knows—weeks earlier I'd helped out the drag queens by stepping between them and some big aggressive gangsta-rapper types and calling the police when they actually started punching. Me, calling the police! What a joke. But the Turks understood where I was coming from and didn't hurt a hair on my head. I'd grown up with them. That was formative. For me, and for them. And the drag queens gave me grateful kisses.

When Madonna was gone, she was gone, as though nothing had happened. That's how things were then: I'd have an experience that would have caused a scandalous uproar in my normal state of awareness but any possible uproar simply dissipated into nothing, whether I'd appeared in handcuffs or had sex with Madonna. Besides, I didn't tell anybody, or only weeks later, soaked in whisky in some newly churned-up bed. The experiences were intense, but without consequences. Every day was like a reincarnation, and a newer and sharper stimulus was required to pacify my consciousness. Whatever had happened the day before was set aside like a war recently lost.

3

Just the word *bipolar*. It is one of those terms that displaces other terms because it supposedly gets closer to what it's naming, and reduces any discriminatory aspect. Camouflaged euphemisms, where renaming is designed to remove the stinger. In the end, the old term *manic-depressive* fits much better, at least in my case. I am manic first, then I am depressed: it's very simple. First comes the manic attack, which lasts a few days or weeks for most people and a year for a few; then come the minus symptoms, the depression, total despair unless, of course, it dissolves into numb emptiness and amorphic gloom. This phase can also last anywhere from a few days to two years, depending on the case, or even longer. I, for one, have drawn the year-long ticket. When I slip down, or fly up, it's for a long time. I can't be stopped—in fall or in flight.

The word *bipolar*, which has had a certain positive impact as a new name for the illness—including a number of other, milder forms of the disease—has also to a certain degree become a technicality that tempers its true, catastrophic meaning and makes it fit for the files: the disaster becomes a consumer-friendly *terminus technicus*. The word is so limp that some still don't know what it actually means. And this lack of knowledge speaks volumes. The educated middle-class citizen with no experience of this condition hardly knows what to do with the term "bipolar," let alone the illness. Such things are still completely foreign to most people, and profoundly disturbing—but this is not to blame them. The word is cheap, the condition shattering. Here we have those who are normal, who also suffer their neuroses, phobias, and real follies, but are still lovable and retain their nod's-as-good-as-a-wink integrity while over there are the crazies quarrelling with their incomprehensible conditions, impossible to fit into any structure, beyond irony or the use of humour to adapt. That is the fate of the mad: they offer no basis for comparison; they have lost every connection to the rest of society. The sick person is a freak you have to avoid; they symbolize non-sense, and such symbols are dangerous, not least for the fragile construct called everyday life. Like a terrorist, the sick person has dropped out of the social order and into a hostile abyss of incomprehensibility. Cruelly, this person cannot even understand themselves. How can they ever make others understand them? All they can do is accept their own incomprehensibility and try to live with it. Because nothing is transparent anymore, not their inner life nor the outer world. Medical explanations are simply examples created by rationalizing doctors as they try to construct meaning and help the patient over the shock of their loss of self: certain neurons were firing too aggressively, a certain stress was counterproductive. But such ersatz explanations have about as much to do with the actual experience of the disease as a handbook on a braking system does with a multi-vehicle crash. You're at the crash site with the instruction booklet in hand, looking through the technical sketches for the wrecked parts in question while the victims are splayed out in front of you. And you don't find a thing. The facts are beyond explanation. The crash was not foreseen during the construction. It would probably be best if people suffering from a mental illness—if they even survive the bout—had themselves sedated once and for all, and simply spent the rest of their lives vegetating, without further reflection or pondering. They've pretty well lost everything anyway. Taking an active interest in their disease and trying to analyze it is stressful, painful, and dangerous.

I have become the subject of rumours and stories. Everybody knows something. They've all heard about it, they pass on true or false details, and anyone who hasn't heard gets a short, whispered update. It has seeped into my books. They deal with nothing else, but try to conceal it dialectically. This can't go on. The fiction has to stop (though of course it carries on secretly). I have to reclaim my story, I have to let the causes emerge through exact descriptions of the crashes even if they don't show up in the technical drawings.

Causes, causes, causes. Take ten therapists and you'll get a hundred causes. The one constant is so-called *vulnerability*: literally, the capacity to be hurt, which refers first and foremost to being susceptible to mental illness but can be read as a kind of thin-skinned-ness, a hypersensitive sensibility that quickly turns everyday life into an impossible burden. Too many perceptions, too many glances, and too many thoughts about what others might be thinking constantly taken into consideration, so that the perspective from outside dominates the inside. Someone who suffers from this kind of vulnerability cannot enter a public space, for instance, a theatre, or a bar, without feeling extreme stress at the social tensions that might be present. Many possible dangers lie in wait. Small talk becomes a trap door, the glances other people might exchange turn into attacks, fragments of conversations impinge on your concentration, just the fact of standing around plunges you into deepest loneliness. The vulnerable person has to make constant efforts to overcome this weakness unless they want to disappear completely into their sociophobia. Unable to resist, and confused by all outside factors, they avoid the social and unlearn how to deal with it, if they ever knew. Or they're driven to desensitize themselves with alcohol and other drugs. Which starts upsetting the neuron balance, gradually overturning it. Maybe. Maybe a reason, maybe a cause.

Sixty percent of those who are bipolar have a history of substance abuse. Does this abuse stem from the disease? Or does it bring on the disease? Or is the relationship reciprocal? It's difficult to know. When you shine a light on causes, they become see-through and threadbare. They provide explanations that may serve to placate both yourself and others, if only in regard to so-called traumas. But they are not really useful—mere simplifications, magic spells, or just plain lies. The medical world is still feeling its way forward by trial and error, as it has been for centuries. Its medications are usually random solutions. Psychology is stuck in the feedback loop of cause and effect. At the end of the day, not even yawning has been explained.

All I can say is this is how it was for me (and this is how I hope it will never be again). But it's impossible to pin down what is cause and what is effect, and which aspects of one's behaviour have not been affected by the illness at all. And so I have to tell the story to make you understand it.

1999

1

"Something's wrong."

We could agree on that. Lukas meant it differently than I did, but he was smart, and kept the phrase so general that I could agree with him. So something was clearly wrong. I thought—with the world. He thought—with me.

A rooster crowed. It was a silly toy in the shape of a rooster that made metallic noises when you moved it. Andreas was holding the plastic thing in his hand, and letting it crow over and over again. It was probably pretty harmless kidding around, a takeoff on what had triggered my paranoia: a signal, a sign, crowing, yes—it's for you. And it's nothing. Just kidding around. Wake up.

The first night of my mania was over. I could hardly remember it. I'm certain I'd managed to sleep, even with all the frenetic action. I'd probably also calmed down over some beer, which doctors actually call self-medication. That's how quickly judgments change: one minute you're a slacker getting drunk, and the next you're a sick person self-medicating.

My friends were quite helpless, sitting around me that morning at the kitchen table. They had never experienced that kind of thing, ever. There was a story of a law student who'd lost it the day before her final exam and identified herself on the phone as her grandmother. I listened to that one, I was receptive to such stories. Now I was about to become such a story myself. And my friends sat there and didn't know what to say. Their glances ranged from furtive to annoyed.

Knut was the only one who, in a swell of emotion, tried to break through the curse, the helplessness. "But none of it is true!" he shouted red-faced into the silence. A good, almost great, attempt that is undertaken far too rarely. No doctor would utter such a phrase; on the contrary in their talks with patients nothing is ever challenged, everything is just noted down: "And so everybody knows you?" "Yes, everybody knows me." "Since when?" "Since, I don't know." "Ah, yes." "Ah, yes." "And do you hear voices?" "What?" "Voices? Do you hear them?" "Yes, yours. Quite clear." "That's not what I mean. Other voices?"

If you answer yes, it automatically means "schizophrenic"; a no doesn't mean anything just yet, it leaves all the options open in this multiple-choice operation that never queries the patient's answers and just nods approvingly. Such practices doubtless have some long-standing justifications: people who suffer from paranoia are seldom persuaded to abandon their convictions. But I sometimes wonder if an interjection from a person of authority, a simple negation of the crazy ideas—perhaps just in passing—in a casual remark, might not be useful. "By the way, what you're thinking about isn't actually true, but..."

Knut at least made the attempt. Or rather, the attempt burst out of him, uncontrolled, Knut being the hothead he was, and living up to the stereotypes that came with his red hair.

"But none of it is true!"

I remember how, as I stared at him, a pause occurred

and reality—the normal world of the day before yesterday, the more or less stable order I knew—shone through. I remember how for a few seconds, while the others were awkwardly silent, I simply believed him, was able to believe him. Maybe my ideas, which consisted mainly of emotions, were simply not true? Maybe they were wrong. They were constantly changing anyway, had no central core, no anchor, no shape. But in that case, what was true? And what exactly did "it" refer to? Something had happened, otherwise we wouldn't be sitting there. And very soon the moment of possible clarity faded away, and I tied myself up again in a knot of confused conjecture. Only on the inside, not uttering a word.

Because fear kept me silent. Not only were my thoughts too wild and new for me to express, but fear and shock made it virtually impossible for me to open my mouth. I was still too shaken, too exhausted from the day before. I was struck dumb with panic, and no longer knew up from down, inside from out. I just stared helplessly at my friends, then lowered my gaze back to the tabletop, where it stayed. The grey sky appeared as a dull reflection on the varnish. A hot mash filled my head. These were the same old friends, the same immediately recognizable, trusted faces and minds, but everything had changed; a great strangeness spread between us, a frontier of the unspeakable. The rooster crowed again. I was completely alone.

The day the whole world went away. You have to imagine it like a fast-forwarded adolescence, a sudden upheaval of all values and opinions, opening eyes that are immediately blinded, the loss of innocence, but not over a period of years; it all happens in a day, within hours, almost in the blink of an eye. The whole world is suddenly structured differently than you thought. You haven't yet seen through the principles and laws but they are painfully present, reaching right into your edgy nervous system. As a novice you stumble, you argue, you rave, and you say nothing. You don't understand, and fall silent. And then you start yelling, defiant and scared. What you once knew no longer exists, everything is strange, you yourself are an alien in an alien world. Consciousness has lost its very grip.

"People are acting so strange," I stammer.

"Of course, they're acting strange, because *you're* acting strange!"

Yes? Another brief moment where a return might be possible, a glimmer of normality, the leverage of a healthy human mind. True, I'm behaving strangely, I ran all through town accosting people I didn't know. Weird, what's going on? But then you think: they're not strangers. They know me. Since when?

There was no explanation, and Lukas caught me up again: "Something's wrong." I nodded; that I could agree with. Something was definitely wrong, basically wrong, wrong to the very core. This core needed to go to hospital, not me—which is what my friends suggested. They finally convinced me to start by leaving my apartment.

2

I walked down the streets feeling high. The concrete seemed to give way under my feet as I went along, but as soon as I focused on this feeling it disappeared. Everything seemed artificially lit up, the facades of the houses looked like stage sets. The atmosphere felt loaded and sharp, a swoosh swept in from a distance, you couldn't hear it, you could feel the pressure, not the sound. Even the air seemed to have turned into a surface. Yesterday there were no boundaries between me and the world, it was total dissolution in the euphoria of signs; today I was completely isolated from everything around me. It was hard to find my way in the streets, though I actually knew the area perfectly well. But there was no more actuality.

In a Turkish restaurant called Deutsches Haus we had lentil soup and kofte. It was my first food in days. I had trouble eating because I felt I was being watched, I was afraid the other guests were looking at me. When a camera team arrived to ask about people's reactions to the earthquake that had hit Turkey the day before, I felt like puking. Of course I took the camera personally, even when it was not filming in my direction. In my mind, someone in authority wanted to prepare me for my new role. Knut had to laugh at the absurdity of it all; he'd noticed right away how the camera team whipped up my paranoia.

Monologues burst out of me. A friend of Andreas and Lukas had joined us and his horn-rimmed glasses as well as the pert confidence he exuded immediately riled me. I'd found a new enemy, although he wasn't hostile. He was simply talking about some host family that had offered him a banana for an upset stomach. It had helped him. I must have been talking about how often I'd thrown up over the past few days and the banana story was probably meant as advice. This "banana" was probably one of the first words I was able to understand without assigning it a secret message, but I torpedoed his testimonial, threw in a few crude comments, and even went on to call the Turks having lunch at neighbouring tables "burek pimps." Andreas snorted and said, "Spaz," which made me grin. But it felt like I was only performing this grin, like I had performed every single grin so far for my entire life. Then I was quiet again, deliberately trying to ignore the guy with the horn-rimmed glasses while at the same time keeping the camera team under observation and ordering my disorderly thoughts, which were running hot. I took the earthquake, whose dreadful effects we could follow on a small TV screen, for a piece of theatre. For one long moment I felt like crying again, and then an exceptionally loud and quite untypical burst of laughter surged up because a joke told by the guy with the horn-rimmed glasses, whom I suddenly liked, struck me as absolutely hilarious. Again, I felt like I was high on dope, but sharper, more precise, overexposed, and without the heavy dullness that smoking pot usually brings on. My eyes were seeing everything, and nothing.

That evening I was back in my apartment, alone. I puked three or four times. I had to spew out the signs that filled me to overflowing and were poisoning me. But it was no use. They stayed inside me. Everything stayed inside.

3

INSIDE   "it's a breeze"

2:32 p.m. Every death I die is one more betrayal of the truth. The surprise party for Lukas ends with me being admitted to a closed psych ward. When you go for a piss, the door to the bathroom is left open. A normal place, like any other, a *not new* experience. Weird. I'd like to be writing it up from *outside,* and not from in here with the outcasts. Who wrecked these people?

Dr Mabuse: rock on. Lost it yesterday. No door handles here. I'm locked in. Herr Melle (also "Mehle") is not allowed out today, could you bring back some cigarettes for him, Herr Noeres. Herr Noeres is *reliable.*

3:12 p.m. A plot—by my friends and friends of friends.
On Thursday night they organized a secret meeting
at Lukas's place, shared information about me: who
knows what exactly has been going on, where is this
leading?

Magda was there too, apparently: betrayal by Magda.
It's a little hard to understand why some people turn a
joke into an illness, when it's still a normal old joke for
you. That's how a cool flyer project that had nothing
aggressive about it got me locked up in a closed psych
ward. Crass difference between message sent and
message received. A friendly gesture turns into a stran-
glehold. What are the mechanisms driving this?

Don't cry a river for me.

11:30 a.m. Here too, I play a leading role, just with my
presence. Grotesque. So I play doctor, and offer advice.
Even when I say nothing, I am the centre of interaction,
everybody's friend. Yesterday a crusty old general, von
Gustroff or something like that, wobbled over to see
me after lunch, a smirkingly cheery volunteer led him
to my table step by tiny step. He mumbled a monologue into my ear that consisted of recognizably lucid
and grammatically correct sentence structures but was
impossible to understand, something about the seating
plan at dinner, and the potential though not absolutely
necessary discussions we needed to hold about this
plan, we could call a general assembly of all patients,
he apologized for interrupting my dessert course with
this proposal; then he excreted a few more word fragments, whispered mutterings, from his almost rigid
mouth. I said I understood, and thought it was good
(I'm not at all mocking him here), and I told him I'd be

considering this. "Herr Gustroff, we're leaving now," the volunteer says, friendly yet determined, and for the third time, we'll say thanks and goodbye now, and Gustroff announces, quite clearly, that we will doubtless cross paths again soon.

I am reading: Robert Gernhardt's *Lichte Gedichte* (Light Poems), Rainald Goetz's *Abfall für alle* (Garbage for Everyone), a comic book series called *Preacher*, Catullus and Horace, a little Wittgenstein. Wittgenstein is too crazy for me right now. Luhmann extra: *The Society of Society in Society.*

A gang around me in the smoking room. End of these notes.

5:32 p.m. Yearnings yesterday. Not necessarily, in fact not at all, for sex, but for two specific female persons, their skin and their closeness. Nothing more. Don't understand. Why am I so alone? Who is that supposed to help?

So sad.

Still, if yearnings were always fulfilled, the yearned-for would disappear. End of the relationship: clinging unfreedom. Crap.

Tea and cocoa in vast quantities, and I've been smoking like the madman Annoying Olaf (more about him later), filter cigarettes. The romance of the crazies, being something special: the root of all madness. I, on the other hand, make every effort to say *I am a normal person.* Take that! And stop staring at me. I say I'm building a house from the way you look at me, and you—you can just go ahead and build your own world. Whenever someone comes into the room, I'm the first person they look at, intuitively. I see streaks before my eyes, which is why I want nothing more to do with F. Having sex with her was already voyeuristic. Let's see how he goes about it, our little porn star. *Lost Highway* was nothing in comparison. Now she's a lesbian, that was to be expected.

Not open—closed.

A closed circle—the entire ethics. The new perspective is not new.

And the nasty comments are not deliberate, in their irony, their distance, their laconic chuckles. I always feel that it's mean. Why are there no urinals in the bathrooms here? We're all men. This is the closed psych ward for men, or did I get that wrong?

9:02 a.m. The Che-Hippie-Goa-Guy is playing Massive Attack and Funny van Dannen for me (but not saying so). A hunk with a drug psychosis is drawing crosshairs on the board, someone else has turned a sketched penis into an ornate plant. I, on the other hand, absolutely refuse to put even one chalk mark on that stupid board over there. That's not where I perform.

The druggie hunk asks me for a urine sample. I say no.

Shoot him in the eye: chalk, board, crosshairs (sketch).

11:00 a.m. SAUNA, SO NEAR AND YET SO FAR

1:45 p.m. Just a quick question: how are you supposed to maintain even the slightest bit of trust in your friends if the tiniest, admittedly maybe weirder-than-usual, action is secretly reported to the conspiratorial cabal and in the end used against you. In the end? What does language say? "End"—which one? whose? what with?

This moment of alienation, a blitz of time in consciousness—

10:34 p.m. Disturbance this evening. The general calls everybody together and makes a lot of noise about a fire policy. He is looking for his pants. They're all nuts.

Magda came by. Nice. The others too: Konrad, Lukas, Andrea, Isa, Knut, Andreas: a short visit. Played a board game called You're Bluffing. The director general gave me a hug. Annoying Olaf (more about him later) says, "You have bouts of anal in you."

But the director says, "Can I call you director?"

We do it like the military: lights out!

Lights out in the bed of the directorate, that's how we do it, poets peter out, loud and fluent:

"Seven friends" is how he calls me out—

"And nobody cares" (me playing You're Bluffing).

5:47 p.m. Contact Ulrich Janetzki, right away next month. Smoking and watching. Waiting to be le(f)t out. Sorry, wasn't doing anything bad. Me good. Good and sick, in institution. What's the reason? What's the reason?

6:34 p.m. POSSIBLE TOPICS FOR FINAL PAPERS AND DISSERTATIONS
Wittgenstein's nakedness
Sleep in literature
An analytical philosophy of literature
Missiles in the literature of the 20th century
Paranoia in the literature of the 20th century
Pynchon and the oldest systems program of German
    Idealism

Disgust in Brinkmann and Goetz
Drastic drama—Sarah Kane and Werner Schwab
Critique of psychoanalysis
Cyberpunk and neurobiology
Bernd Alois Zimmermann—time as sphere and
    depression
Mind the surface: creathief writing
ha, haha, haha
haháhahahahá

0:01 a.m. Guard, automatic?
In exile

4:03 a.m. sleepless
Excursion into 2008
Unfortunately, I don't see you the way you don't see
me

(From my notes, September 17–21, 1999)

4

Your first stay in a psychiatric ward is usually traumatic. You've crossed a line, the doors close. Michel Foucault is no use in here, there's no reciting the discursive or plain old power relations and mechanisms of exclusion: the theory and history of madness are of no concern to anyone. You're confronted with praxis here, no, you are part and parcel of a praxis that eludes any subjective influence. So all ye who enter here, let go all images of self. You have arrived where nothing is right anymore. You are greeted by screams and slurping noises. And a loaded silence, the kind of silence that develops when silent people have been waiting too long for something. Except that the patients aren't waiting for anything in particular. At most, the next dose, or their first leave, but more likely a distant deliverance. They're just waiting. This is a foreign, thoroughly regulated world, a world that is uncanny right down to its bureaucratic details, located right next door to the normal-sick world, just one building over from X-rays and a floor above Orthopedics.

You suddenly step into the realm of madness, its smells, visions, faces, and phenotypes. I remember an admissions interview with a robust, manager-type doctor, who I quite liked in his masculine pragmatism. I probably agreed to being admitted for fun, out of curiosity, or to calm down the friends sitting there next to me. They'd been working on me, and they promised to visit regularly. I was not completely with it, still hadn't realized that I'd lost my mind, which immunized me somewhat against disagreeable impressions. I viewed it as a research visit, complied with a chuckle, and maybe even laughed about it secretly. Over the next days I sometimes addressed the other patients as though I were the doctor in charge. There was nothing traumatic about it; that came later, with the depression. I was just too psychotic to recognize what was really going on.

Just have a smoke, I thought, and headed down the long corridor with the fake dark marble flooring. In the smoking room you could feel the routine of years, heavy with time. Newcomers like me either got a feeble greeting or a suspicious stare. I didn't say a word, and smoked with the others, in this pigeon coop of nicotine and intense paralysis. There was aggression in the air. People came, smoked, and went, the door opened, the door closed, nobody said much. After two cigarettes I got up, stalked off to my room, and sat down on the bed. My roommate was plucking away on his guitar, an amateur, after he'd told me he was a star.

I recognized his self-aggrandizement immediately, unlike my own. I listened for a moment, wondered how such a twisted misperception could develop, jumped up again and hurried across the corridor, had a look at the day room, checked out the board games and books, felt immediately bored, and swaggered back to the smoking room. In five minutes I had covered the territory of the next few days.

5

Contrary to the statement of a head doctor who ten years later would become a not-very-helpful reference after I had spent months in his clinic and only seen him once, the manic does *not* remember every detail. It is quite the opposite: they remember very little. Mania, writes Kay Redfield Jamison, a professor of psychiatry who suffers from bipolar disorder herself, is a merciful disease as far as memory is concerned. She says mania wipes out most memories. Which is largely true. But I don't know if this should be seen as merciful. The lack of access to your actions and experiences represents one more, retroactive, loss of control, which next to all the other losses of control that acute bouts of the disease bring on may seem rather mild but it further undermines the patient's already weak-ened identity. Personally, I would like to know what I did during the bouts of mania, and as completely as possible. I have access to short fragments, particularly crass or drastic events, and also unspectacular moments, encounters with people, bits and pieces. But much of what I know about my behaviour I have only heard from others. Others know a lot, I don't. Still, some images and situations are so sharp and so garishly present that an attempt to reconstruct the connecting pieces does not seem completely hopeless.

6

1999. It was a wild summer, and a somehow depressing one. I was out often with my new friends enjoying the euphoria that alcohol and music sometimes brought me. It was the era of the bar scene: going to Cookies and the Eimer club and following Kunst und Technik. It was the era of Berlin, which held an almost greater promise than university had, the promise of the metropolis that had been calling us for years, with its chaos, its clubs, its beat, and all the spirit assembled there, the culture that kept us moving, the excesses we were looking for. I say we, as if I were speaking for others and not just for myself; but I was one of them, one of us. I was part of it, and I drifted along through night life and every day, through new, hot books, and newspapers and ideas, through the still young internet, the seminars, the city. I saw myself as part of something.

Finally there, finally on the go—but right from the start a lowering feeling that constricted my chest, my breathing, my gaze. I felt like a slacker, just hung around sometimes, drank, but was still a hyper-diligent student. How did that work? It just did. A long-distance relationship that had started off with a lot of romance quietly fell apart. The days grew paler, the U-Bahn rides longer. The Free University was a genuinely cold machine in an enchanted, faraway suburb, Dahlem. The seminars became burdensome, but I kept at it and read everything, and sometimes felt the same old craving. I worked hard to counter the inertia, the dejection, and was already quite disoriented—among the anonymous crowds outside and in the inner continents of ignorance that grew ever more monstrous the more I studied and read. I wrote a seminar paper on Robert Musil, obsessive and precise as though my life depended on it, but after the professor made an admittedly flattering comment wanting to know where I'd learned to write like that, I just let it go. Why did something like that slip away? Why had I even put out such an effort? The anonymity of the university finished things off; the students' fear of contact was quite absurd, especially in the rather elitist department I was in. And as the most fearful, I was soon left completely to my own devices.

I'd hang about, listless, not knowing what was next, and then resisting this low point, I'd leap up and head out into the streets, wander about aimlessly, through supermarkets, in search of Punica Oase or some other *product* that could *deliver* something, wouldn't find anything and would slink back to a silent, chilly apartment. I'd sit there at the kitchen table, make a sandwich I'd only eat half of, and try to get back into whatever I was reading. Which was still possible then.

This state of affairs had existed before Berlin. It had already been there in my childhood, my youth, my adolescence: a persistent feeling of being off course and always having to overcome the gap between the world and myself, not only for a couple of hours or days, but fundamentally. And every time I felt enthusiastic about something, the hateful other side would show up, blank, stale, empty. If something made me happy or gripped me, it soon died, grew foul and objectionable. Profusion inevitably gave way to emptiness.

Already in Tübingen. I started university there in 1994, fired up and impassioned by a great will to learn and with such energy and momentum it must have put some people off. For high school graduates, university presents a promise. Finally, the young mind can pursue its own interests, unbothered by an often rather frustrated and therefore constraining group of teachers, far from family, and in my case, quite dysfunctional working-class conditions. Recreating yourself in your studies, finding your way, increasing your knowledge, sharpening your skills—those were my goals. I wanted to be an A-student and live my own *Bildungsroman.*

I chose to take ancient Greek in a class that was scheduled at eight in the morning with the theology students in the Protestant Seminary, and I *crammed* in the most old-fashioned way. And the day went on from there, to seminars, the library. Inexhaustible depths opened up, and stuff I had earlier considered weighty literature I now read for relaxation between blocks of theory. At least that's how I saw things, and I read Hans Magnus Enzensberger and Hermann Broch in my breaks. I was enthusiastic about the teaching and inspired by the unconscious joy of still being invisible, still being free.

Around the end of my first year, a few friendships with students in analytical philosophy developed and alleviated my isolation. After a Friday evening video we'd go out to the Depot, a house club in the industrial park, and shake our bodies free. Some of the tracks set off a euphoria in me, *everybody be somebody,* that I loved.

But things soon took on a greyer tinge. *TEMPO* magazine ceased publication, and that had a surprising effect on me. I couldn't believe the sales clerk, and felt that the magazine's demise put an absolute end to my youth. I found the seminars more difficult and more boring; my motivation decreased but I kept on attending. I could see something basic was wrong. Deep down I was sure I was not suited for university, or even for life. The daily grind of getting up, getting dressed, heading out, Greek, the seminars, ingesting food, library, home, sleep, bored and frustrated me. From my time in boarding school I was used to being in a social group of people with similar ideas, however different they were as individuals. There had been a certain dynamic that carried me along and that I even helped mobilize. This dynamic no longer existed. My new life, which was supposed to be starting, wasn't really getting off the ground. The supper I ate at my writing desk didn't taste good. I avoided the kitchen on my floor of the student residence, for fear of the business and education students who considered me suspect and ignored me. I was slumping, things felt stale, not even two brief love affairs helped. In the third semester I dropped Greek, started skipping seminars, and instead spent time on a hillside overlooking the city, studying the roof-tile-red misery from above, this overheated Swabian nest of idealistic thought, or I went straight to the movies to remind myself of what I really wanted to do: create fiction, not theory.

Why was my mood so black? How had I ever landed there?

At night, at Hölderlin's grave, I would realize that I was just *making it all up* in the most perfidious and complicated way. Then I'd strike out to the twenty-four-hour shop, buy cheap Le Patron wine, with which I doggedly tried to stimulate my reading and writing and resist paralysis. But every morning, every day, began with a new despondency that didn't dissipate till evening. Tübingen was one year at full throttle and one year choked with doubt and despair.

Later, in Berlin, I realized that even though we had not been introduced by name, I had encountered a real depression.

7

In the weeks before I was committed, I'd fallen slowly but surely out of touch with myself and doubtless with others too. I remember how the heat affected me that Berlin summer, and how helpless I felt at the post-novel-writing void in the first months of the year. The novel was titled *Saturday Night* and was set on a Saturday night. Five characters live through an unhappy party and an almost microscopic analysis reveals the false foundations of their young lives: tragedies on the edge of a dance floor. It was a riposte to the rampant pop literature of the time, using the same background but set in negative rather than positive tones, writing depression and resistance rather than contentment. Over a period of a few months I stressed those four or five hundred pages out of myself and onto a nicotine-yellow computer screen, and was as exhausted as I was happy at the end of it. It was done, and I hoped it was good. I sent the manuscript to a few publishers as well as to the Literary Colloquium Berlin. I was ready for the avalanche.

But nothing happened. The summer just went on and grew thinner. The fact that reactions to literature can take a little time did not mesh with my natural impatience. And the boost that writing the book, which was never published, had provided now produced consequences that I struggled with. I still felt the hectic tension from the effort I'd put into the book and the joy I'd drawn from it. But there was nothing to calm down my agitation or direct it toward peaceful productivity. My perceptions closed down, my mood slumped.

I'd been in a hurry. Benjamin von Stuckrad-Barre, my age, had brought out his first book a year earlier, and then Benjamin Lebert, still a kid, came along with a hit about a boarding school. I liked this stuff and followed and read everything without envy; yet I kept pressuring myself. Wasn't I the one who should have long ago brought this moment into cultural awareness with all the tools of my art? Wasn't my perception, my language missing in this landscape of discourse, text, and thought? Of course I was being extravagant and vain, and I was aware of this, but I was still unable to let go of the fixed notion that I needed to write *the* novel. In fact, I'd only been to university in order to read and understand enough to acquire the refined tools with which I would lay out the abominable beauty of our time. While I was still arguing with Derrida and using Aphex Twin to get through the nights, the first bloggers were getting ahead of me.

Today you can laugh or comment ironically about the exaggerated self-assessment of this young eccentric, which is what I do, but despite all the skins I have since sloughed off, it is still rather embarrassing for me to acknowledge that this is how I was, this is how I *may still be*; it's as embarrassing as some of what I am writing about here. The excessive tension, the ambition, the all-or-nothing attitude, the exaggerated and therefore quickly disappointed enthusiasms were probably early indications of what was awaiting me. The restlessness, the self-imposed pressures, the delusions of grandeur that would often, within days, turn into an inclination to drop everything, the total inertia and profound inferiority complex, these fluctuations were typical of a manic-depressive temperament though not yet of the disease that bears the same name.

8

It starts with an excess of emotion. No, it starts earlier, with a period of incubation, monotonous days and weeks of vegetating in cotton-soft indeterminacy, a dumb sort of dimness, comparable to the proverbial "calm before the storm"—a time I remember only vaguely because it was pretty vague. Contours of thinking and feeling go blurry, perception dulls, reflexes are lame. In some obscure way, I

only partially exist, a ghostly, marginally conscious appa-
rition, already almost gone. This paralysis is preceded by
restless efforts, followed by extreme exhaustion, squander-
ing strength and self. More alcohol, more writing, less sleep.

If I ask friends and acquaintances today what they saw
before my first bouts of illness, and in which situations they
already suspected *there's something wrong*, they provide
examples of quite usual behaviour on my part, but behaviour
that is just a little more aggressive, more stubborn, more
radical, that of a monomaniac. I latch on to some specific
project, a piece of drama or some unsuccessful blog, and
talk about nothing else, totally preoccupied by distant oth-
erworlds, while not being completely present. I hardly see
the person I'm talking to and react impulsively, with sharp
exaggeration. And then I backtrack, rein myself in, censor
myself.

Effort, extravagance, exhaustion, paralysis—and then
the explosion. Manias seep secretly and slowly into many
a patient, and gradually intensify from hypomanic, overwrought, and hyperactive phases into the classic frenzy.
This was not my case. Apart from the condition of paralysis already named and described (which should also be
considered part of the disease—but along with what else?),
it takes only seconds.

So, it starts with an excess of emotion. A shock flashes
through the nervous system, cascades of random emotions
shoot downward and come swilling back up. You feel a total
lack of restraint. Your skin grows hot from within. Your
back burns, your forehead is numb, your head empty and
at the same time overflowing: floods of neurons. From one
moment to the next shapes of thought disappear, re-form,
and re-establish themselves, rush away from the usual centre. Your brain hurtles off without its owner. What's up? But

this question only flares briefly and can't be considered in the flurry of emotions. And then your gaze gets snagged on some detail, the sky turns into a diffuse threat. Then the first thought arrives, and building on that, the second and the third, and the thought processes quickly frame— thought by flawed thought—a structure that provides an explanation for the excess of emotions. And you cannot see that this structure is based on completely false assumptions and crazy hypotheses. It just keeps building, skittering on, unrestrained, and like a demented handyman it builds a makeshift shack of thoughts that serves, momentarily, to bed the excessive emotions in a provisional, short-lived set of explanations that won't be valid even the next day.

It starts with a minuscule, mutating detail that proliferates like a madly fantastic structure, constantly changing, mor- phing like a Steve Cunningham animation through the most multifarious incarnations. Details accrue, settle in, become hinges, support beams, are rejected and exchanged. A con- stant, ongoing process is under way, a process of building worlds and destroying them. Madness is a process, not a con- dition, and it can last hours, or weeks, or months. Or a year.

A few vague basics survive all the changes. The psychotic can always reach back for them. These basics are usually par- anoid. *I* am the focus, and *they* are out there somewhere, con- spiring against me. But the basics remain vague, which is why the psychotic can keep calling them up in many variations.

That is how feelings find their rationale. And this ratio- nale, as worm-eaten, poisonous, and sick as it is, sends you off on a trip to heaven and to hell.

9

My mutating detail was a tiny sentence on the internet. My school friend Lukas had brought me into a lively group of law students who liked to party and who I spent weekends with. One day gave me a call: he was onto something that might be fun. Oh yes, and what was that? It was access to ampool.de, a literary chat room project on the internet that was insufficiently secured with a weak password, and that I'd recently become aware of in a short article in *Die Zeit*. I'd been following the sluggish activity there ever since. Although interesting writers like Judith Hermann, Rainald Goetz, and Christian Kracht were billed, there was hardly anything going on. Lukas figured we should use the password he had cracked to remedy the situation.

Lukas was a mischievous trickster, but not to excess, and he was also a nerd. His humour was both charming and self-deprecating; he went about a little dreamy and awkward, and with a mocking kind of intelligence that, like his body, moved in jerky, nervous twitches, and didn't seem quite mature. He'd grown up in a strict Catholic, but very open-minded family in Bonn, in a house whose back door was never locked, as though there were no such thing as a thief in this world (and of course, they were never broken in to), and this had provided him with a rock-solid view of the world, full of trust in other people. Lukas was keen on education, but not pompous about it, self-conscious and modest, a pianist, a Dostoyevsky fan, and a computer expert who had run a fairly chaotic PC-repair service while we were at school, which at that time, in the early nineties, was pretty unusual. I often benefited from his knowledge, like when my stone-age computer that had no graphics had to be fitted with an internet connection.

"Now what," he'd say. He'd be at the computer, I'd be standing behind him. We often stood or sat like that, to figure out something digital. You have to reach into a kind of rascally vocabulary, to talk about the way Lukas was then: an old-fashioned trickster who liked finding ways to "bug" the teachers (though we didn't talk like that ourselves). We'd just finished being the kinds of high school students who'd burst into a friend's oral final exam to offer both examiners and examinee a cardboard pack of cheap white wine called Domkellerstolz—Pride of the Cathedral Cellar—plus some orange juice as a refreshment, only to be scolded by the school principal: the *Matura* exam was actually about being mature, were we aware of that? We'd been highly skilled at those kinds of actions, and now, four or five years later, we couldn't quite abandon them.

"Not sure," I said, a little uncertain.

"Oh, come on. Let's write something using their names."

"Okay."

And that's what we did. We had Rainald Goetz mark his return from vacation with an eager "HALLO WORLD," and Judith Hermann warble out a mindless triplet "cross-eyed, cross-eyed, cross-eyed" as a response to a "double chin" entry by Christian Kracht, and we let Moritz von Uslar wax delirious about Luhmann's "problem of the observer" in his supercool oral-texting language. Then we posted all this, had a quick laugh, another beer, and headed out to join friends and hit the clubs.

10

For a time, I believed that if I hadn't gotten involved, I would not have gone mad; without this dumb schoolboy prank, that soon tangled me up in a meaningless parallel world, I would never have plunged into the first abyss. But that is probably not true. I was susceptible, without being aware, and the madness was lurking, waiting for the right moment, which I was innocently and actively bringing on by overextending and overexerting myself, through isolation and excess. It would have happened anyway, the way it happened again later, triggered by something else. Still, I can't help asking the age-old question, *what would have happened if.* Or in this case, *if not.*

11

There was a bit of turmoil at ampool.de, people got excited, annoyed, laughed, applauded, or were snootily silent. Lukas and I had set up a fake dialogue between a couple of the chat room members, and then when everybody found out, we came clean and apologized, which led to a riposte that I couldn't help reacting to, and that inflamed the situation anew. It was a fight, it was fun. Some of the chat room members who occasionally commented, announced that from now on and under these conditions, they would remain silent. That really got on my nerves, but I'd already been taking it all far too personally. I started filling the stagnant pool with my own effusions, about life in Berlin, the summer, the slacker mood I was in, the somewhat hysterical aspects of my life. I mixed stuff I'd read about with experiences I'd had, and enjoyed myself in the process.

But my responses weren't normal anymore. I worked myself up into a me-narrative that soon became like the monologue of a confused now-I'm-the one-that's-speaking type. In one of the back rooms of my brain a small guilty conscience kept smouldering away. I stubbornly wore myself out with those contributions, dissed a considerable number of stars, dropped a phenomenal number of names and waited for reactions.

Precisely this yearning for attention, these expectations, that I was already pumped up with from the unsuccessful novel, those hopes and the internal feedback loop, were about to shred my head. I had no inkling of what was coming, though. I'm not sure how long I spent on those posts, three or four days maybe, then Lukas opened a counter-page, the "Realpool," where we continued writing; meanwhile I was convinced that I had to "save" the project. Beer and sleeplessness did the rest, and to top it off I fell in love with one of my co-writers if that is even possible in this mediated way. It was grotesque.

I kept on posting way too much, in our Realpool, in the guestbook, I clamoured and nagged, I whined and rejoiced, and gradually other people started coming out of their hideouts and writing about their lives, in tones that ranged from shy to triumphalist. From my overwrought perspective, it was a movement: a generation, silent until now, was finding the words to express itself, which fired me up even more to give it my all. I overheated and exhausted myself, already somewhat manic, thought of nothing but posting, producing torrents of words from a life stuck in neutral. Lukas, who probably felt that something was about to give, and who had already said it could "all be a little friendlier," wanted to end the whole affair with a final chat. We drank, we chatted, we shot the breeze, and finally ended our self-aggrandizing mockery.

When it was finally and really over, I missed it, probably as a pressure release valve, and an opportunity to engage with others, regardless of how stylized or cartoonish that was, and also as an egotistical performance I'd found intoxicating. I lay around for a few days as though I'd been punched in the head, dull inside and at the same time painfully on edge. Some people missed my posts. I did too. After the novel, the pool-action had provided the next hit and I was left feeling empty and raw. Something had burst open, in front of everybody. I felt unwell, wanted to turn things back. I felt shame. For a few more days my blustering interventions fuelled conversations among the anonymous as well as the named posters; I watched that, feeling exhausted, wanting to get back in and somehow correct the megalomaniac impression I seemed to have left. But it was too late. It was over, and I had to hold back to not totally overextend or make a fool of myself. I lay there like a sad little pile of ash and didn't know where to go next. The sun hung, unmoving, in the sky. Then came that Thursday.

12

Exhausted brain cells are dozy and dopey, lying fallow, but something is brewing. An imbalance has slid into view, but no, it's been there all along, probably a genetic gift that is now being confronted with overexertion and effort, and made worse by alcohol and work. The nerve cells are packed in tightly to the thalamus and the frontal brain stem, far more tightly than in the case of healthy people: studies mention one-third more neurons. The thalamus bundles the sensory perceptions and sends them on; the brain stem controls the level of activity of the entire organ. Both functions will soon be running wild; sensory perceptions will crackle, and levels of brain activity will soar quite out of control … Piece by piece, impulse by impulse, everything will keel sideways, slowly keel over, in order to then revolt. But nobody knows what's going on yet. Least of all the brain itself. That's why the first neurotransmitters paw the ground with their hooves—they are the messengers that carry information from cell to cell: serotonin, noradrenalin and dopamine. Normally they conduct the signals and ensure the activity of the organ as well as rewards and expressions of emotion. They have long grown tired of being mere waiters. They are increasing in numbers and planning a hysterical riot. Soon

they will overrun the terrain and hurl demands across the
room, against the walls, and into the guests' faces, pulling
the entire establishment to the left.

That's when the brain's metabolism boils over, and the
person loses it.

13

I was staring at the screen. The letters were starting to
dance gently, maybe the pixels were fluttering in the heat.
I was reading. Unbelievable, what was going on! My computer was weak with age, and so the page came up slowly
and in fragments. But the individual sentences that gradually appeared were sending special messages into this brain
in particular. Just the fact that it was taking so long for the
page to load set off a dull suspicion that they'd blocked the
page, that Lukas had contacted the webmaster and they'd
decided to wean me off the site by sabotaging the system's
speed. That was a first vague gust of paranoia, an ember
that would ignite my whole thought system in seconds.

My eyes caught on one specific sentence that could be
read in various ways. It was about some kind of vehicle at
the Brandenburg Gate, a bike or a car or a tourist rickshaw,
I don't recall which; at the same time, I felt there was some
unspoken reference to me. How was that possible? What
was going on? The words were about the vehicle and about
me—an ironic comment, an elaborate metaphor? It threw
me into total confusion, but I couldn't quite believe my
interpretation. Why was I suddenly being referred to? And
were there other such hints and signs? I concentrated, read
a few more sentences. Now the other posts, too, seemed to
suddenly refer to me, or *also be meaning me*, in a cleverly perfidious way that was not explicit and could always have been
denied. For instance, a reference to a rather sinister guest

at a party made me wonder if I was meant, if I was being described, or if the writer wanted to tell me something about myself via the web. Or in a discussion of an enthusiastic article, my own enthusiasm seemed to be included, or the enthusiasm I had actually triggered in some people. This paranoid reading strategy took over in minutes, I couldn't help but relate everything to myself, tentatively at first, and then compulsively. And too often, it seemed to fit. Whether the topic was a walk in the woods, or a hard drive, or a stop in a café—the ironic way people wrote about these things always left a vacuum with just enough room for me, semantic vibrations that made me tremble in synchrony with the tremors in the fields of meaning. Every word could mean me, the adjectives, the nouns, the verbs. How did they create this effect? How did they manage to be talking about me without talking about me? It frightened me, and I panicked. What had I done, and what were these people doing to me?

Sure, I'd been hoping to step into the public eye, make my voice heard, loud and clear—but not like this! I realized that my uncontrolled intervention, overwhelming them like a force of nature, was now producing consequences I could not fathom. They (they? who exactly?) were overwhelmed, had to deal with it, digest it, and get rid of me by indirectly negotiating around me. Some of them pelted me with dirt, others praised me in flowery language, and one woman fell in love with me. But I couldn't be sure. Maybe I was interpreting it all wrong? Scraps of reason came back, and suggested I was having the thoughts of a madman. Really! A madman. The reactions that were flying around before my eyes were just my imagination, weren't they? Take a deep breath, I told myself, keep calm. It's just your damn narcissism, foaming over the edge of the glass! But I couldn't keep calm, I was too upset and shaken by cataracts of emotion

I had never experienced before. My heart was pounding.

I had to move, I leaped up, stared at the wall where tiny bubbles of paint were visible. Those bubbles must have a purpose. I'd never seen the wall this way before. What was it hiding? The comments of all kinds of people over the years shot through my head. *Directional microphone* someone had said, *underground catacombs* someone else. Were there cameras in my room?

I flung myself down on the worn leather couch and looked out the window at the sky. It was cloudy. And pulsating? I jumped up, stepped out onto the massive balcony, and stared upward. Nothing, only grey. The house across the way, inhabited by squatters, stood there, unchanged. Was someone moving at the window? Hadn't all the windows just been lit up, and now as though by order, hadn't they all been deliberately blacked out? But it was daylight.

As though someone were watching, I threw my arms around in dramatic gestures that acted out being overwhelmed, but at the same time conveyed an ironic comment on what was obviously a crazy situation. But nobody was watching. Or were they? I kept gesticulating, gripped my head ten times in a row, and hurried back to the computer. There it was, it was all there, right there! And my name too, sometimes in code, sometimes unscrambled. But I was no longer interested in those arrangements. It was the other kind of talk, the talking-around-corners that electrified me and that I now had to decode to even begin to understand what was going on. I started going over the earlier posts, examining them hastily, checking for anything I might have missed. And of course I was able to twist and turn those sentences in any direction and come to all kinds of conclusions. How long had this been going on? To enlarge my sample, I even went back to posts composed before we "broke in." But there was no reference to me, thank god. The secret code seemed not to have been at work there. But wait a minute—hadn't the long silence of the chat room members, back when the action began, been strange? Wasn't this silence an indication that people were content at the certainty that I would finally and surely arise from the legends? Which legends exactly?

Hey, look at that! They'd cast exactly the right people to attract my attention. Those were all well-known tricks and ploys, weren't they? Or did the stubborn silence of these popfreaks just express an enormous fear I couldn't yet understand? Why the silence? I sensed something, and followed up, going hectically through all the entries from before my arrival. Even the old words I hadn't influenced suddenly began to shimmer and point in my direction. What was that? Had they been waiting for me? Was this website a trap? Were elegant degenerates just waiting for their redeemer? Or their hangman? Or what?

One thing was certain: an internal shift had taken place in the language, but I didn't know exactly what it was, how far back it went, when it had happened, which posts had already been manipulated, who was secretly having fun, making fun, or just afraid. I couldn't figure it out no matter how many calculations and comparisons I made. I understood both everything and not a single word—a "deviant hermeneuticist." I giggled to position myself. But I felt electrified right to the tips of my hair, in orbit already, lost to normal comprehension, gripped by a diffuse semantic madness.

It is not easy to graphically describe this kind of madness, because there is nothing graphic about it. It is an internal displacement of language and discourse, a dissolution of meanings and the connections between them, and the vectors flitter, rotate, and point cheerfully in all directions, and keep turning back to the madman. Every aspect of language—and what is not language?—is twisted and unruly, the signs have been ripped off their moorings. Nothing means what it means anymore, but everything also always means "me."

In a state of absolute alarm, I read, and pondered, and kept clicking. Other pages now seemed touched by the same effect. The most diverse remarks by politicians and celebrities had something hectic about them, and there were always secret messages in them for me—for me, right here at this writing desk. Gerhard Schröder talked about my coal-cellar childhood, Joschka Fischer advised moderation. It was hard to take. Was it a worldwide plot? And if the internet was talking like this, what would it be like out there on the streets? I suddenly felt paralyzed by fear, but I had to face the situation.

The excess of emotion was enormous. And these feelings had to be coming from somewhere. They couldn't be overpowering me from out of nowhere. They were there and they had their reasons. And I was hot on the tracks of those reasons.

14

I have to pause briefly at this point. I have told the story of what happened on that devastating day quite often, in my books *Raumforderung* (Room Required) and *Sickster*—but in a controlled, literary, abstract way. I have even taken paragraphs or longer passages and reprinted them because the narrative struck me as so appalling I couldn't and didn't want to produce yet another version—like someone who has been traumatized and keeps repeating the same sentence because the story behind it (the event, the disaster) can't be told. Doppelgängers and recurrent figures pervade the works I have already written and published. So why describe this Thursday, this day of confusion, and the first bout of the disease again? In order to banish the doppelgängers forever? Maybe. But the real reason is much simpler: if I want to report on that day years and now decades after the fact, then I have to take one more close look at it.

Besides, the context, the purpose, and the style of this version are quite different from the earlier texts. I am not concerned with abstractions or literature here, effect or drama. I am concerned with a kind of truthfulness, a concrete account, or at least the attempt at such a thing. This is about my life, in essence about my disease. So the original outbreak has to be part of it. I want nothing to be qualified, exaggerated, exoticized. I want it all to be open and visible, as far as that is possible.

15

A party! Of course! They were organizing a party. For me, probably, or for us, for everybody. For Lukas! For all of those who felt anonymously connected—silent for so long—and had now found their way back to language. We would fall into each other's arms, talk, drink, dance. Scales fell from my burning eyes; somewhere in Berlin a party was being organized, it might already have started, with a stage and a sound system in place, stacked beer crates, only I was missing and eagerly anticipated. The signs were friendly. A treasure hunt was about to begin. I couldn't miss the big find. I quickly dug out the street map, shouldered my backpack, and stormed down the staircase, which applauded me. The way would find its way on the way.

I raced down the street, throwing my legs from my body, no, that's not right, they threw themselves into the din. The cars swooshed past as though wanting to cheer me and pull me along. Everything was out of line, out of place.

I'd never seen the worn-out Vietnamese guy look so soulful, and I bowed to thank him for the food he cooked for me now and then. He raised his eyebrows, acknowledging my thanks, and I was able to carry on, totally happy, without ordering food. I roared down Devastation Boulevard, trying to overtake the cars while the shutters on my left winked at me, motionless. They were arranged in such a way that it was obvious these houses were faces, but I was only now able to see that, even as I rushed by. The cars sped up. In which of these innocent vehicles might there be a hint about where the party was, and what form would that hint take? All-knowing, they zoomed by. I couldn't control myself at the lights and stormed into the traffic as I thought about that Czech film director who once claimed at a conference in Prague that Germans would all stop on red like a bunch of electroshocked cows. He was so wrong! Electroshocked, maybe, but not on red! Just watch me charge into your stupid red! At the next light I ran into people I'd just seen at the first light, and I laughed at how perfectly the scene was arranged. How quickly someone had brought them in, behind my back, to overtake me. Or were they tricky doppelgängers, extras from some agency specializing in twins? When I saw they were just waiting for me to laugh so they could laugh, I had to laugh, so we could laugh together. And that's what we did.

Letters of the alphabet were actually hanging over the city. Who was their creator—me? I rushed on toward Mitte. I was on a mission, a huge mission, though I couldn't have said what it was. Where the hell were my friends? The signs? Oh, the signs would show up soon enough—or were already spread around everywhere, I just had to learn to decipher them. Actually, posters were already sending intense messages, but the codes were set too wide to allow

precise narrowing. You dumb coked-up ad agencies! Your
messages streak by without effect. I had to reach back in
time while I was moving forward in space, and I tried to
remember what my roommate had said at lunchtime. He'd
mentioned a few addresses in Mitte he'd visited, or what
exactly? And one was in Novalis Street. Novalis? Novalis!
When Numbers and Figures ...

Waves of panic washed through me but I was able to
let them pass and ebb off. Phrases flew through my head,
ads and proverbs and quotations. They pulsed through
my brain as fixed expressions, then fell apart into shorter segments, then syllables, and finally mere phenomena
that besieged my inner ear with noise—persistent techno
rhythms I couldn't ignore. I got into an S-Bahn, was surprised at how quiet it was, said something into the silence,
and got out again. In Novalis Street, books in a store window suddenly turned into threats. They got mixed and tangled up with everything I'd written in the last weeks and
months. An alphabet of letters stormed toward me; objections, accusations, threats smashed into my head. What
had I done? What was happening? Had I challenged the
heavens, was I wrestling with angels? Was everything turning hostile? I looked around, turned once around, whirls
of lights, echoes from the depths, decreasing gravity. The
physical vertigo came out on top of the psychological vertigo. My mood tipped completely. There was too much to
calculate, to watch out for, it was all a huge *too much* bearing down on me. Where could I go? Where?

16

I spent the whole day running around the city like that, and
my enthusiasm gradually turned into panic. The street signs
and notices became monsters, as shimmeringly threaten-

ing as the sentences on the internet had been earlier. The net had expanded and enveloped the city, everything was changeable, ambiguous, and unbelievably new. I had never seen the signs or the world in this way, but this was probably how things always had been, only I hadn't noticed it. In the end, every message always also meant me, and I was still looking all around. It made me dizzy again and again. The notices and lit-up ads started mocking me. If there was a blindfolded woman, she was there to make fun of my earlier blindness. An arrow with an oversized *WHAM!* meant: *We've got you! You're cornered and caught, up the creek, enough fuss from you, it's over!* I fled from these signs and at the same time sought them out. How could I not? They were all over the place. Ordinary street names started turning into rude jokes. The city map didn't help. Suddenly I was afraid that I was becoming a Nazi in newly destroyed Berlin, and dissolving in tears I told this to a cyclist, who pointed at a light and said, "It's green." Then he rode on with his family, a little flag on his carrier rack. What was that supposed to mean: *green?*

I ran on through the city and the city had gone crazy. Signs and images clutched at me from every corner. I avoided them skilfully whenever I could, but I had no real chance of getting away. The crowd kept hitting me hard. They'd been normal old slogans, and notices, orders to buy and street signs that didn't mean anything special. Now they were showing their truly gross faces and reaching for my sweaty shirt collar. The air alone was a poisonous cloud. I was a video game avatar being shot at, but what with exactly? Shot at by signs? Weren't they the same as always, as yesterday? Was there something different? Yes, I thought, and ran. *Everything* is different. The pixels were flittering in my face.

I would have laughed if I hadn't been in such a panic. And I did laugh, or there was laughter inside me, but like an echo. From the bunkers under my feet I resonated upward as laughter. The city's maw was quaking. It wasn't deep drilling, it was a surface explosion. I was making the city tremble, and at the same time it was roaring through me. It was no longer clear who was setting whom into motion. I had no skin, no barrier. Everything was beating down on me as destructively as it was, as it had truly and always and essentially been. It not only beat down, it diffused and radiated through me. The two of us, the world and I, were dissolving into each other, suffusing each other.

Why had I never noticed this before? Why didn't other people notice? There they were, the others—*hallo!* I approached them—but as if at a secret sign, they would disperse, not obviously, and not in obvious haste. What was wrong with them? If I asked them something, they didn't answer, or made some gesture to fend me off, or pointed to a public telephone. Some so obviously pretended to be deaf that that, too, must have been a message. I kept running, heading for the Spree. Fewer signs there, I hoped, fewer people.

Something had overturned, something had tipped over onto the city and then into my life, and all in the space of moments. Where had it come from—this disturbance, this menace? It was bigger than the city, bigger than the country. It was as big as all of history; it was universal. I had to resist, even if all I could do was run, flee. And that's what I did. I ran and ran, panicky and still lightly euphoric. And then again, my tears came, uninhibited. I couldn't flee, impossible. It was everywhere.

When I reached the Spree, I briefly caught my breath. But even nature had lost its innocence. The water was messaging differently than before, the glimmers of light on the tips of the waves perturbed me. I considered jumping into the river. A great guilt was burdening me. Whose guilt was that? Mine? German guilt? Original sin? I didn't know, I just felt it bearing down on me and I broke down. I was on the bridge, seeing myself drift by below as a corpse. A draught came from out of the darkness. I clutched on to the handrail as though it were a ship's railing in a wild, stormy sea and counted things: one, two, three, a hundred. I couldn't go on.

A soft wind picked up, probably coming out of hell.

Then I ran off again, my legs like two torn film strips, flapping and rotating in the emptiness.

17

The hours rushed through me. When I asked about the party in the house across the way where the squatters lived, I ended up with a bloody forehead. "So what are their names?" a woman with thick glasses barked at me when I knocked at her door and asked for my friends; her partner, a cross-eyed punk, grabbed a broom, broke its handle by smashing it into the floor, and slammed it into my head. There was blood, but the wound dried up. It was getting dark outside. In the Kastanienalle I asked two guys about the party I hardly believed in myself anymore. They laughed, maybe at me, and said it sounded good, they'd like to get invited to a party like that sometime too. I pressed on through Mitte, Prenzlauer Berg, Kreuzberg, into entrances here, and down streets there. A long piece of blue wool thread led me to a parking lot, but the only things waiting to be decoded there were licence plates. Memories shot through my brain, chaotic and wild, fragments of sentences, of pictures, echoes of things that suddenly meant something different than before. Everything was moving, nothing was solid or within reach. The trucks roared past me in a war against the bicycles, exactly the way the papers had described it just the day before. Yes, "When the Trucks Go Mad" that was how *Der Spiegel* had titled the article and now I was witnessing the truth of this headline that screamed of madness. Truck upon truck thundered past me, raising clouds of dust in a hellish racket. What the newspapers shrieked about on a daily basis was, in fact, true—exactly true. Worn down, but still electrified I hurried home and listened to my answering machine. Only chaotic messages. An architecture student I hardly knew wanted to talk to me about Paul Virilio and the speed of rearmament, as we'd agreed a few weeks earlier. Pardon? I pored over letters left unopened and understood nothing. They were saying something different from what they seemed to be saying—wasn't that so? As a student of literature I was more than cognizant of the metaphorical aspect of things, but these metaphors seemed to be global and downright vicious. The simplest sentences told lies. They only pretended to refer to the realities they represented. Numbers were codes, sentences ciphers. Even invoices thought and spoke sideways. I lay down on the floor.

When my roommate's girlfriend came back, I tried, in tears, to get something out of her.

"But you know, don't you, Antonia? You know."

"What do I know?" Her frightened, narrow eyes didn't understand.

"You all know, don't you?"

"What? What do we know?"

Yes, what exactly? That was the problem. If I'd known, I would have told her. But I didn't know. I knew nothing. I was the one-who-didn't-know, the new one. But she knew, she had to know.

"Antonia! You've got to know!"

She looked at me in dismay, didn't know what to say.

"I'm going to call Lars, okay?"

"Okay."

"Okay."

I fled to my room and combed through newspapers that had been lying around for weeks. How long had the internet action lasted? Four days? Two weeks? I'd missed virtually everything that had gone on outside during that time. Was it true the press had reported on me, and in that sarcastic, allusive way? An article on "retro-futurism" in *Die Zeit* had attacked me. It was of course written in a mocking tone, literally sneering at me. But I found the accompanying illustration absolutely lovely. I even felt like I had never in my life seen anything lovelier. In fact, all the newspapers displayed good aesthetic taste; the editors must have been making special efforts in recent days. *Die Zeit* beamed at me, as did *Süddeutsche Zeitung* and even the *Berliner Zeitung*! Only *Der Spiegel* kept shouting. And the grumpy old *Frankfurter Allgemeine Zeitung* was still so rigidly stuck in its senility, I almost wanted to find it cute. Eyes fluttering, I ran through the articles. Joachim Kaiser had published an article in *Süddeutsche Zeitung* about the new inhabitants of a digital realm, accompanied by a sketch of a jittery cabled-up freak in a jittery cabled-up world. So he'd reacted to me too? What did he say that was intelligent? Later. First I had to figure out what the general mood of the papers was. But in my hectic approach I couldn't define any general mood; I kept getting stuck on details that concerned me. The advertising in particular was making fun of me, crude and crass. I turned on some music to drown out the quiet I didn't trust.

So the papers were in on it. They'd also started talking in that many-layered, dishonest, but perhaps well-meaning way. Everyone was pulling on the same rope, and I was the only one who hadn't got the joke. Since when? A suspicion came over me. I glanced over at my bookcase. What if...? I leaped over to the bookcase, opened one book, and then another one. Then still others. The more I read and the more I leaped around in them, the more the sentences tilted their gazes toward me. So the books had been in on it too, right from the beginning? I didn't want to think about it anymore and shut my eyes.

18

The drama that a first psychosis unleashes is considerable. It is an unimaginable, all-encompassing blow that flings you into outrageous orbits; for your friends and family it is a total tragedy. Suddenly, out of nowhere, someone they know goes crazy, literally crazy, and in a far more precise, more real, and more embarrassing way than is ever shown in books or films, goes crazy like one of those wild-eyed derelicts who yell at the traffic, and turns stupid, foolish, weird. Out of nowhere a friend becomes a stranger.

Out of nowhere?

Manic-depressive illness is usually assigned five different causes: genetics, changes in neurons, life circumstances, the already described basic condition of vulnerability, and finally, personality. These categories merge and blur. But they offer a sort of direction, a way to understand; even if only one of them fits, and never completely, it still affords a hypothetical template with which to compare the chaos via four or five structural parallels drawn from other cases, and so to extrapolate explanations. I remember the long-distance phone call my friend Cord made, completely dismayed by my new condition, and how he regained a bit of his composure after the doctor told him it's all a question of neurons. That was something he could live with; it turned the change in personality into something objective and physical. The reasons were physical; the doctor had shifted them into the realm of bones and nerves, basically like a broken leg, and, as a person, I did not yet have to be given up for lost.

19

The gene for bipolar disorder has not yet been discovered, if it even exists, nor is there any genetically determined pattern, as in Gregor Mendel's work, that might help you predict who will fall ill and with what degree of likelihood. But both bipolar disorder and schizophrenia have some genetic causes, and the symptoms often overlap and occur in the same family. Even more frequently, those who have bipolar tendencies will find unipolar depression—pure depression, in other words—in their family tree. That is my case.

My family is no stranger to psychic frailty. My mother's father, they say, suffered from phases of depression that were never clinically treated. It was not done at the time and would have run counter to his military discipline. Although, from a child's perspective, he seemed to swallow a large number of pills every week, there were probably no antidepressants among them. Officially, he had heart and blood pressure problems. He died "upon retirement." And only offhand remarks were ever made about his dejection and melancholy; they were nodded into non-existence.

My mother has a long, and very clinical history of depression, one of my aunts as well, but milder. So there is something about the genetic material, at least on my mother's side.

As far as I know, my father's side has no history of psychological anomalies. As far as I know—since that side has hardly been present.

20

The whole world was gone. Everything was being dragged away. No earthquake could have done more damage. It's just that this earthquake was different: it was taking place inside me, and the destruction, all-encompassing as it was, was silent. Nothing stayed the way it was, and yet from the outside everything seemed the same. Language no longer had an anchor but people continued to talk, quite normally, though they were strange, completely distant. I would have had to learn this new language, but how could I, without a grammar book or a dictionary, and so I was left to myself, to my weird self, that was in the process of dissolution. Layers of stories and counterstories monstrously coated my thinking, no sentence told the truth, everything twitched and flickered. Smoking ruins were all around me, yet, at the same time, in me alone. It was pure horror.

The days flew off in all directions. Paranoia blossomed, proliferated in every corner, became omnipresent, and I eventually settled into it. What else could I do? Every now and then panic would turn into a defiance I had to shout out, then into a euphoria that carried me to the highest heights. For a short time it was cool to be the messiah. I no longer felt my body; I had magic powers, was in tune with the laws of nature, heard the rings of Saturn hissing round and the musical cadence of the spheres. I reckoned I had now intuitively understood mathematics and saw myself cosmically connected to everything. Then again, the greatest terror: although I was standing there, naked and exposed to the chilly breeze of the universe, nothing changed, and I, the chosen, broken creature, simply did not know what to do. Again and again I had to break through the centuries-old prison of time, history, and teleology where I believed I was, break out verbally or with a quick twist of my body, or with another mad dash through the city, or with strange emails sent to foreign institutions, in which I tried to present things from a funny, satirical angle, but was really only greedy for new signs about what in heaven to do. The TV ran non-stop in the background as it had throughout my childhood, and when I took a close look, almost sinking into the screen so that my hair crackled against the glass, I could see how sorely the souls of the speakers and news anchors were thirsting for attention, how horny they were, their souls more so than their bodies. Late-night host Harald Schmidt, on the other hand, was a step ahead. He had installed an invisible friend at his side, whom he mocked mercilessly, and to whom, in a mean twist, he had assigned the moniker Horst. Asshole! I laughed, but I knew I was constantly turning myself into this fictional friend, this Horst. How could I help it? If I did nothing, everything around me, right down to the Gaza Strip, would only get worse; if I played the fool, I was at least still present, working on a solution. This unbelievably dreadful fate, its dreadfulness not yet fully realized, justified any kind of behaviour. In fact, it was appropriate to display a radically different behaviour than before, what with this new awareness of my capacities and the responsibilities now burdening me. At the same time, I wanted to shake off these responsibilities and regularly held my own private carnival in order to get free. I drifted through the city, made inappropriate jokes, posted something somewhere, and no longer slept. At home I ran endless loops of the recent and paranoid-plot films *The Game*, *The Truman Show*, and *23*, hectically read books in no chronological order: Samuel Beckett's *The Unnamable*, Ingeborg Bachmann's *Malina*, *Heinrich von Ofterdingen* by Novalis, Augustine's *Confessions*, *Gravity's Rainbow* by Thomas

Pynchon, and Goethe's *Elective Affinities* as well as Plato's *Phaedrus* and Orwell's *Nineteen Eighty-Four*. Time was out of joint, and I had fallen out of it, out of time, and landed in the cracks. Did that happen to everyone who wrote? If I considered some of the biographies of crazy people, then clearly yes, it did. If I let myself think in this way I could see that the mould I was now being fitted into had been created long before my time. The early Romantics were murmuring in my ears about their despairing search for the god to come, and Goethe, too, was responding in sonorous and compassionate tones about some kind of world citizenship. How could I have missed all this before? Kafka addressed me directly, in his god-fearing and at the same time bureaucratic manner, really spoke directly to me. I was the Steppenwolf, I was V, I was Oskar Matzerath and Godot. And the dead dictators in history were beginning to yell in my direction too.

Newspapers, which I bought in huge quantities, fell to pieces before my eyes. Then I would storm off again and party, greedily and without inhibitions. I had to forget myself and all the rest, if only for a few crazy minutes. Actually, I only wanted my old life back.

It was true: something was wrong. Quite seriously wrong. My friends worked on me, sometimes as a gang, sometimes one by one, taking turns, they conferred, came to decisions, devised strategies. After I had doggedly resisted all their efforts for three or four weeks, they finally managed to persuade me to go to the Charité hospital. The Charité was a piece of history and carried a certain status. Charité was Rudolf Virchow, Ferdinand Sauerbruch and the anatomical freak show with the crippled *Tin Drum* fetuses, that I'd already found fascinating.

As I said, I saw it as research.

21

The psych ward basically houses a hodgepodge of failures, who are thrown in together and react in accordingly
wild ways. Depressives with schizophrenics, manics with
borderliners, amnesiacs with suicidals and addicts—all in
the same space. Of course there are regular blow-outs, of
course people yell, cups and plates fly through the air, and
frustration and madness burst through. You're jammed in
with everyone, in one ward of a hospital, whether you're
actually the king of Germany or the angel of the damned.
The king has to learn to wait patiently before he can dictate
new dispatches for his subjects, and the angel doesn't care
because he's beyond time and space anyway. Or you're just
a zombie, without resources and basically finished with
life, wondering why you're still there.

Which reminds me of Harald, a good-natured, skinny
guy, who'd shuffle through the ward with a Ping-Pong pad-
dle in hand, uttering monologues soaked in spit that were as
friendly as they were beyond comprehension. Only sometimes he would talk about his father, and almost cry, and
that's when his speech suddenly became very clear. Once
he lost it and burst into an angry rant at one of the nurses, which was all the more disconcerting and surprising
because he was normally so kind-hearted and friendly. This
rant was also about his father, and he wished him nothing
but death, but you could see in his still-gentle eyes, shad-
owed with sadness, that he actually missed him terribly.

I spent four or five days in the closed psych ward of the
Charité. I'd landed there because there was no room in
the open wards, at least that was the official line, which I
still accept today. It was all new to me, it was even partly
pleasant, mainly because I didn't see myself as a genuine
patient, I was there only as a temporary visitor. The new

environment and the medication distracted me from my own paranoid ideas; they didn't go away but they were less urgent. My friends visited every day. Sometimes there were eight people assembled around me in the smoking room, which particularly irritated the patient who I called Annoying Olaf. He was right in the middle of a paranoid psychosis and exuded an almost electrical form of aggression, a bearded, slovenly man with glowing, light blue protruding eyes ("Hitler bulbs" is what I wrote), that brazenly stared at me and the others as he smoked in nervous silence. Sometimes he would utter words that came out of some unclear line of thought. When he asked for my name, my answer triggered quite a turmoil because, as he shouted, a man with that same first name was responsible for his being in the closed ward, and this other Thomas, Thomas Anal by name, and a therapist by profession, was an asshole, as his name indicated. And further, this "slimy back-door therapist" kept sending him new and nasty messages, via the "anal canal." But nothing personal against me, he said, it's just a name, just my name. Then he sprang up and left. Running into him was very unpleasant (and of course we were constantly running into each other in this overcrowded ward), because he was so wired and kept trying to make flittering eye contact, in the corridor and the smoking room and the dining room. The fact that in later phases I must have made a similar impression on people sometimes disheartens me completely.

I took my pills, without knowing why. I considered them placebos or some kind-hearted type of drug that made my brain giggle. I felt calmer, but I didn't ascribe this calm to the supposed medications; it came from being cut off from the world, from the asceticism of not having access to information. For at that time (and to some degree still)

I was an information junkie who continually exposed himself to every possible media, with the radio, the internet, and the TV running at the same time while I rooted through three freshly printed dailies, trying as hard as possible to decentre myself. So a few days of seclusion, a few days free of signifiers, and being in a "safe space" could only have a positive, calming effect. Perhaps I would even get to feel my never-before-encountered centre that was such a topic of discussion. Once, something did start seeping in, however, as I was watching a TV report on an explosion in a fireworks store, and I began drawing the most diverse conclusions about what this case of arson had to do with me. But I quickly forgot them again, and instead remembered the astonished but tempered reactions of the other patients who mumbled to themselves or made knowing, dismissive gestures.

I felt calmer, wrapped in protective padding and with an invisible helmet on my head. It was the exhaustion from my first bout of overheating neurons and the medication that dimmed me down. The world was muffled, the paranoia had turned my thinking inside out and stunned it. I was calmer, yes, but also skeptical: where was I exactly and why, and wasn't this just an enormous self-deception designed to assuage my friends? Slowly the realization grew that I was not in the right place, here among these crazy, damaged people. The arson in the fireworks shop had reminded me of the conflagration outside, the real events and revolts, the furor of the signs in this inflamed world, and I was certain there was a task for me amidst all this chaos though I didn't know what it entailed. The hospital didn't fit with what I wanted to be and stopped me fulfilling the duties that had been imposed on me from afar. Because I was there by choice, I could discharge myself, even against the doctors' advice. And that's what I did, returning to the apartment, which my roommate, who'd wanted to move out anyway, had in fact already left. The silence hummed.

22

So the illness I suffer from is manic depression. In clinical circles and increasingly in everyday life, it is referred to as bipolar disorder. This rather limp and—not only from my perspective—rather trivializing (for others a less-stigmatizing) new term was introduced in order to better describe and differentiate the various disorders: bipolar I, bipolar II, cyclothymic disorder, rapid cycling, and mixed forms. Bipolar I is classic mania with subsequent depression, and usually strikes more than once; in fact, a patient can suffer several bouts of it over their lifetime. Those who are ill with bipolar II first suffer a depression, then hypomania, then another depression. Hypomania is a lighter, weaker form of mania, during which the patient feels uncommonly strong, alert, cheerful, and productive, is up early in the morning and in a good mood, without seriously screwing things up the way manics do. (If the depression weren't part of it, hypomania would hardly be a problem.) Cyclothymic patients have the same symptoms as bipolar II, but weaker, though the bouts come more often. In rapid cycling patients the frequency is even higher and may reach four episodes a year, with highs and lows that can be pretty acute. In mixed forms of bipolar disorder, symptoms of mania and depression can appear at the same time or with very short gaps.

I fell ill with a form of bipolar I, the classic, heavy version that Emil Kraepelin, a psychiatrist of the late nineteenth century called "manic-depressive madness." Both mania and depression are fully present. My particular version of the illness is apparently unusually drastic, some call it "nuclear," because the manias and the depressions last uncommonly long, and the manias are accompanied by paranoid psychosis. So when I refer to mania this usually includes psychosis, which leads to a considerable, delusional loss of reality and even to hallucinations. While the average length of time for a bipolar I mania lies somewhere between two weeks and two months, I have so far survived three bouts that were all much longer, and each one longer than the preceding one. In 1999 it was three months; in 2006 a year; in 2010 almost a year and a half. The subsequent depressions lasted equivalently long and were just as agonizing. The one thing that is certain about phases of mania is that depression follows. The more violent the mania, the more profound and tenacious the depression.

They say manic depression is one of the ten illnesses in the world that lead to permanent lifelong handicaps. It is relatively common; between 3 and 6.5 percent of the population falls ill with some variant of the disease at least once in their lives. The number of unreported cases is high: about half of all cases of bipolar disorder are never diagnosed as such. The causes of the disorder are biological and neurological, but it manifests as a psychic illness, with bizarrely transformed experiences and behaviours. Emotions run wild, everything is perceived and acted out more intensely, and this intensity ends in real madness. The sick person feels far superior to others, celebrates their new consciousness, and is full of enormous energy. They tend to be wasteful with all resources, whether these are spiritual, intellectual, or financial. Total lack of inhibition rules— sexually, the manic tends to excess, intellectually to extravagance, emotionally to extreme fluctuations. The ideas and plans they develop by the hour are unreal, their patterns of behaviour are erratic and extravagant. This can result in a great creative push but it can also flop into nothing. Their attention flickers and they can't see the forest for the trees, they focus on twigs and bits of bark, then notice the forest again and smash into the trees. Love gets worn down in a series of violent, chaotic, and sometimes overly strong impulses that are momentary and unpredictable and can lead to brief affairs with people who would have been of no interest to the patient in a healthy state. The manic dresses ostentatiously, moves restlessly and hectically, gives in to shopping madness, sleeplessness, and an unstoppable urge to talk, with wordplay and jokes that can hardly reflect how ludicrous their shredded thoughts in fact are. At the same time, manics present themselves as enthusiastic and high-spirited, which is why it is often difficult to diagnose the condition. They fall into debt and ruin. If their mania is accompanied by symptoms of psychosis, which in earlier taxonomies was seen as schizophrenic but is now seen as an always possible aspect of the bipolar condition, then despite all the euphoric highs, mania can turn into darkest paranoia, negative obsessions, and a total, fear-ridden loss of reality. At that point the only difference between schizophrenia and mania is hearing voices—and the frequency of the bouts. Which is why many schizophrenics may well be suffering from misdiagnosed bipolar disorder.

In regard to the pathology on the other side of mania, which is depression, bipolar disorder leads to almost unbearable spiritual suffering, that words such as *hopelessness*, *apathy*, *lethargy*, and *despair* barely express, and quite often—in 15 percent of cases—it ends in suicide, which every fourth sufferer attempts anyway. The death rate is far higher if the disorder is not treated. Then it outranks all forms of heart disease and many types of cancer.

23

The day after I left the clinic I jumped out of bed at four in the morning and was immediately wide awake; it was still dark when I set off on a feverish walk in the direction of Steglitz, pompously reciting Novalis's "Hymns to the Night" in my head. At eight, I landed at the breakfast table of Magda and her sister, which soon had to be cleared since, unlike me, other people were still attending university. I marched on to the outer limits of the city, and then physically weary, wondered what in the world had happened to the world. But it also felt good to recklessly toss back to the world some of the excess energy I'd loaded up over the years. Whenever too much emptiness developed, new stimuli, new provocations had to be conjured up, whether they were actual—face to face—or virtual because that's where my texts had gone viral, where they were being copied and sent around in the thousands, no! the millions, that's what I imagined. The chancellor was reacting to them, as were Kate Moss, Maxim Biller, and everybody else, very personally. At the ZEDAT, the university computing centre, I posted something on the web and then, over the course of the ensuing minutes, watched how people in the corridors of the institute and in the streets of Dahlem were reacting. Even their silence struck me as suspect. "Dahlem has to burn!" I thought, or said, laughing, then I walked to Lankwitz and back again.

The media was one hysterical reaction machine. Videos were being programmed and designed in such a way that they responded directly to what I posted, even to my actions, the paths I took and the words I said; they fired me up, warned me, told me off, and glorified me, but always commented on me. I was caught in a chamber full of signifiers that were celebrating their own Mardi Gras, with me as the prince, the fool, and even the majorette. Even in my own room I was no longer sure who was watching, who was developing the latest news items or video clips about my posture or the words I'd just posted. I kept checking the TV, spellbound. Everything was live. I sat there, paralyzed by fear, until a sudden fit of rage would blast me free.

Now and then I returned to the seminars where I had to really control myself to make it through that hour and a half. I couldn't sit still and listen quietly anymore. Occasionally I would speak up and start rapping out comments that were far too fast and tended to head off topic, establishing new connections between the early Romantics and late cyberpunk, for example, or cracking stupid jokes, comparing August von Kotzebue, the German playwright, with Hui Buh, a ghost character from a children's book, which made the woman next to me laugh but clearly threw off the professor. The obsessive joking that is typical of schizophrenics and manics had taken possession of my language centre.

In other ways, too, I laboured to organize the chaos into some kind of joke, in order to not slip into total despair. I went looking for the gallery where my former roommate Lars was working. I'd heard there was a new exhibition, something to do with children's books, probably created just for me, the perennial child. The gallery owner was friendly and led me downstairs to the colouring books, literally. This was where you could do colouring? That was what the artist wanted? Yes, she said, and the coloured pencils are over there. But nobody has done any colouring yet! I said. She nodded, and left. She shouldn't have done that, because I now grabbed hold of the coloured pencils and began. For the first few moments, I obediently filled out the shapes with the coloured pencils, adding shading and nuance. But then I went haywire, scribbling chicken-scratch all over the paper, ignoring the lines, using the pencils to wreck the task, while I was still in a way fulfilling it, and then I scrawled the word "DESTROY" across the top in capital letters, which quickly seemed too lame, and so I added another "DESTROY" after the first "DESTROY," sending a better message—in the act of destroying you have to also destroy the destruction. At some point, I got up and left the gallery, not before politely saying goodbye. An hour later I posted a detailed account of this action, full of naive high-tension rhetoric, on one of the internet forums I hung out in because I needed to catch up with and explain the rumour I could feel developing and spreading through the excited media. At home, Lars stopped in for a short visit, and said he'd heard about my action, which he called "impressive," his eyes empty.

I phoned all kinds of people—you could still find most numbers in the phone book—left coded messages, and decoded the few conversations I had back into my paranoid network of relations, then went out into the city with new clues in my head like a video game avatar jumping from level to level, collecting stuff, rushing home, and making more phone calls. I wrote emails to Ulf Poschardt, Jutta Koether, and Dietmar Dath, and phoned Moritz von Uslar. Dath didn't write back, which made me mad at *Spex* magazine and kept me working away at some socks metaphor I'd sent him; Poschardt answered half-amused and half-serious and said he'd enjoyed reading what I sent but it was literature and not journalism; Jutta Koether, on the other hand, told me straight off about the life she was now leading in New York, and in such an honest way that I was oddly touched. She opened up to a crazy stranger, who was happy that she did, but couldn't do anything with it, that's how irradiated he was. I answered in confusion. Moritz von Uslar, whom I actually reached by phone, told me abruptly he hadn't understood the message I'd left on his machine. That's something I understood, and I wondered why he sounded so healthy and sonorous and I didn't. But then, in a matter of moments, this realization flipped into its opposite: his coolness and all the deluded fuss around him had made him sick, and I was the representative of true, flourishing, unadulterated life.

24

We were on the Teufelsberg. I'd been there before but nothing compared with this particular moment, no, with this *momentum*. It was the blue hour, thick with ozone, an ambience that filled the heart to bursting. The twilight made silhouettes soft, bodies see-through, spirits plump. For a few seconds, I felt I could fly. If I were crazy, I thought, I'd try it, I'd stretch out my arms and lift off. Vera and Henrik were standing close by. I could feel them, they could feel me. We were humans, and Henrik pointed to the Le Corbusier house and had something to say about it. I listened and understood. It all seemed very simple.

I am not sure if the metaphors of the Enlightened Ones were having an effect on my perceptions, or whether my perceptions were actually quotations rather than perceptions—or whether I was really experiencing any of this. I believed I was really experiencing it. My hair resembled dendrites. The pressure in my head was gentle but good, my skin sensitive but normal. All set for reception. The triangle formed by the Le Corbusier house, the Teufelsberg, and the Olympic Stadium was laden with history: the pragmatic Bauhaus vision of ornament-free living collided with the monumental architecture of fascism, whose ruins, piled up in the Teufelsberg and crowned with a listening station the Allies had built and that was now crumbling, could be climbed, freeclimbing on the left-overs of the "bipolar world"—and that's where we were standing, inside this triangle, with a light wind blowing from paradise. We gestured to each other, blessed and safe. The tensions of history pushed me further, and away from the others, who I left behind without a word. I climbed up the hill to the station, slipped, and lying on my back, saw the stars up there, which I used to love so much, and which I'd forgotten. They were quietly twinkling, unmoved. The Cold War was over and had turned into a leisure park. This was the doing of young people, I thought, by doing nothing, in glorious dissent, through a collective slacking off in running shoes with holes in them: coming of rage. *This* was the life's work of Generation X. I got up and walked on. The night swallowed me, kindly.

25

A day later (or two, or a week) I was sitting in my doctor's waiting room at the Charité. I occasionally agreed to office hours. A crazy woman was huddled across from me, maybe forty years old, swelled-up and tense. She kept staring at my crotch and twitching on her chair as though in heat. I remained relaxed and tried to send some of my calm in her direction.

As I entered the doctor's office, I suddenly remembered that my biological father, my progenitor as some say—and this thought, this term, made me feel as though I were in one of those countless talk shows that run on TV in the afternoon—that when he heard I wasn't doing well (how was I not doing well? I was big and strong) he'd headed for Berlin in his car but only made it halfway. That's what I heard. I imagined a dramatic, wordless scene: him getting out of the car on the shoulder of the autobahn, in his last throes, making a vague gesture in the direction of a patch of forest, letting his head sink down, exhausted, on the roof of the car. The other cars zoomed past, indifferent. It was filmic, wordless, but highly dramatic. Dead at the halfway mark. At the same time I thought it was a lie. Why should a truck driver not make it from the Eifel to Berlin? Maybe he'd just stopped in at a casino and conked out there, like he used to. I didn't know the man.

Dr Melvin, my doctor, was the most nondescript person ever, you couldn't even say what he looked like. He was all glasses and colourless hair. Drily, he would enquire what I was thinking or feeling at the moment, run through a list of questions, motionless and bureaucratic, withholding all comment. I knew that now and again my concerned friends contacted him. But he said not a word about this. I took him seriously, sort of, just like the crazy lady, who was already gone when I crossed through the waiting room on my way out. They were all playing bit parts.

26

In the manic phase, time flies. Every day hurtles past you, no, actually you hurtle through the days. Impressions are countless, stimuli are garish, sleep units are short. You live with the conviction that you can put everything and everybody under your spell, and every last nerve fibre of your body is imbued with strength, know-how, omnipotence, luck, and then again panic, rage, and guilt.

I started to focus on my enemies, Springer and Daimler-Benz. They were proliferating in Berlin-Mitte, sloshing their late-capitalist and therefore desperate and highly potent poison in all directions, building chunky UFOs and monuments to themselves, and ruthlessly heaving their weight around the centre of the city. I went to the sports section of Kaufhof, looking for a baseball bat. I was briefly distracted by the beautiful, top-of-the-line basketball shoes and pants. Very cool! But no time for frills, and I pressed on, following the lines painted on the floor that were reminiscent of a basketball court. It got even more American farther on, baseball had to come soon. And there they were, the lovely things, hanging in a locked glass cabinet. I had a light sense of guilt, but got a sales clerk to open the cabinet—he suspected nothing and was friendly. I picked up one of the bats, massive, heavy hardwood, put on a professional face as I weighed it in the crook of my other arm, grinned—and so did the sales clerk, who didn't leave my side—and performed a few slow-motion swings with the bat, typical batter swings, moving the bat forward from the back of my neck; the batter hits the ball at the side of his body. A fake look of expertise on my face, I repeated these movements a few times, along with a few light-footed skips as though I knew the sport intimately. At the same time I felt like a Jedi warrior—the bat moved like a slash with a lightsaber, a swoosh through space. I could already see myself smashing through Plexiglas windows, the splinters would fly high after five well-placed blows at the same, now brittle spot, ten thousand shards bursting into the sky which itself would develop cracks to the wail of a Depeche Mode alarm. There would be no stopping me, and no way back. The entire showroom would get it, and I would quickly batter the Mercedes limos on display into futuristic scrap art, a statement against capitalism *and* against art— blow up the cash registers, trash the categories. Then I'd hike over to the high-rise Springer building in my combat boots, capped with my street-fighting cap, the one Susie sent me from London, I would quite deliberately—hmmm, yes, what exactly would I do to the Springer building, how would I shake it up? Would I have to lure the old lefties out of their villas, would they join me and finally consummate that arc of their lives? Blast those reactionaries!

I couldn't think of anything concrete, and the sales clerk beside me was growing impatient. Besides—a baseball bat against a whole high-rise building was akin to using a screwdriver to fight a tank, right? And then I couldn't line up these crude fantasies with the rest of my self-image. Was that really me? Nothing but a *mini-terrorist*? These moral scruples brought on the thought that even my choice of enemies might be clichéd. Hadn't those battles all been fought already? Which battles were left to fight? The baseball bat in my hand went back to being the dead object it was. A laser? You wish! It was more like I was mutating into a dumbass. Ludicrous.

"Yeah, pretty good." I returned the bat to the sales clerk, thanked him, and went off. Then I turned back and bought myself a basketball.

27

Every now and then I would still go out with friends, get drunk, approach girls I didn't know with the name of my internet love, confusing everything with everybody. Every room became a cavern heavy with meaning, populated with unimaginable figures. I was crazy about Magda, for a time, for a longer time, and she responded, let herself be carried along by the torrents of words, no matter how wild or meaningless they were. When she came to see me, I would put on *Fritz the Cat*, a pretty drastic animation of a comic strip that I didn't like at all, but that seemed to be an irresistible tool of seduction with all the dope-smoking and the sex. I was the comic-strip tomcat.

I really liked Magda, but quickly forgot about that and

at some party talked up another girl, whose name I don't remember. She stopped by as well (her phone call coming just after a call from another girl, my internet love, which struck me as somehow planned and weird, a paranoid take, whereas they didn't even know each other), but she couldn't handle my monologues like Magda could. I made her uncomfortable with my purpose-free nattering, and she wanted to get away, insisted we go to the Christoph Schlingensief evening at the Volksbühne Theatre which we'd been considering. On the way, she informed me that I had an "alternative relationship to the truth" which I, of course, totally misinterpreted—not as the aslant, off-kilter relationship that she meant, but as the only correct, good, and truly truthful relationship, the only key that would solve all mysteries. And I began to discuss the various theories of truth—consensual, coherent, image-based, *the morning star is the evening star*—to then set up my own crude hypothesis that provided my metaphoric facts with first deductions. I thought the girl incredibly beautiful.

At the Volksbühne, we stood at the open side entrances to the main hall, and I announced that I knew Christoph Schlingensief personally, as I also knew Michel Foucault, who I thought was still alive. I was in constant communication with them both. I was referring to how we agreed about texts, which was crazy enough, but I made it sound as though we were really friends. And weren't we truly buddies in our struggles against the forlornness and the faults in the system, each for himself but also for the other? The show had started and I was getting more and more frantic, shaping words, twitching back and forth, impulses searing through me like small electric shocks, but before I could shout anything out, she checked me over one more time and said, "I think we'd better go."

And she led me away.

On the rainy walk to the S-Bahn, Clemens Schick, a friend of my former roommate Lars, crossed our path. I yelled out a cheerful, "Clemens!" as though I were his friend. He stopped, and the situation went rigid. He looked at me in surprise, and rather than keep talking, I fell silent. Now he and the girl had to engage in small talk, which neither of them wanted, and their glances revealed that they were both aware of my condition, I know that today. I remember those glances, which I misread then. Maybe Lars had already told them? Or maybe it was just too obvious.

"And what are you going to do now?" he asked, friendly and a little uncertain.

"We're going home," said the girl with an oddly serious look on her face.

Then all three of us nodded, wished each other a nice evening, and we and Clemens went our separate ways.

When I recall this situation, this scene in the rain at the Hackescher Markt, with the up-and-coming actor Clemens Schick there in front of us, and the way I watched the girl out of the corner of my eye as she talked, then the feeling that this illness brings on is completely present again. How weird and inappropriate things are. It puts me in the room next door to reality, a back room I can't get out of—and it all comes back as I remember that short, quite unspectacular, encounter. The image isn't stashed in my memory like a normal image, but like a scene I look at through a windshield sprinkled with raindrops and a steamy interior. I'm there next to the other two, I say something, I say nothing, it doesn't matter. I could yell, we would be just as far apart. They look at each other. What resonates is the impulsive, inappropriate greeting, the way it startles me, and how I brush aside the irritation. *This* particular triad comes up again and again: thrust, withdraw, ignore. Then the embarrassed silence and at the same time the desire to break through all the fakery; the inability to correctly interpret the glances of other people who I know know something. One part of the nervous system is aware of this incongruence and is quietly trembling, but consciousness itself, unfortunately, ignores the problem. There's a tension, like in a scene from a film noir, with attractive, thoughtful people and the intuition that something is seriously wrong. The blue eagle eyes of Clemens, who won't remember the incident; the beauty of the nameless girl, who will never read this account; and the strange dishonesty I hear in their words and that I catch as I eavesdrop on the whole situation, unable to name a single detail of the slanted take, those lies, never knowing where the dishonesty actually comes from.

I am that detail, of course. But I don't know it. The pressure in my head, the filmic rain, the blurry lights. The excess, the absence, in his eyes and then in mine. The care people take in dealing with me that seems to wrap everything in gauze, a behaviour that in similar situations later on will unsettle me much more. The incongruities. Withdrawal, and thrust: the attempt to dissolve the light and the impenetrable auras, those halos in the rain. The fake halos. The rain, the eyes. The futility.

And then the prosaic continuation of the journey. I brought the girl to the station, and quickly wobbled home, listened to ear-splitting music, read a few excerpts from old books and new articles, fell asleep, and three hours later jolted up again and lurched heavily into action.

Years later, the same girl spoke to me on some dance floor and asked whether I still knew Schlingensief, or if in the meantime, or how... and if I'm not mistaken she had a slightly mocking look on her face. Healthy again, I'd forgotten or repressed the incident, but her nudge brought it all back and I didn't know what to say. She smiled and danced away, and I realized that not an evening, not an hour, of my madness was forgotten; somewhere, forever, it continued to make its mark.

28

That's how things went for two or three months. Fixed ideas remained movable. The fact that the so-called millennium was approaching further aroused me. I suddenly understood the hysteria around the millennium that I'd shrugged off as nonsense, and I got infected, since I was obviously one of the sources, if not *the* source, of this terrible hoax. Things seemed to have been under way for a long time; *I* seemed to have been under way for a long time. I'd ponder how long people had known and observed me, trying to establish when exactly the soul of the world had been struck by this accident. I bought the almanacs, popular at the time, for the years 1987, 1983, 1982, 1979, and 1977, as well as various world almanacs, published by Fischer, and studied political and cultural occurrences, recalled the lyrics of pop songs, interpreted and sang them anew. They'd always been talking about me! Advice, reinterpretations, commands, invective—I was getting it from all sides. I was stuck in a tangled coil of lyrics and news, receiving the most contradictory messages in whispers.

Soon the years 1982 and 1983 became the focus. That's when the child I had been so far was turned into an involuntary human experiment. I saw the 1982 change in government in a new light. The searchlight of the world spirit had picked out a little descendant of people from Silesia, located him in a project style housing area in Bonn–Bad

Godesberg where he'd grown up in rather turbulent circumstances, and so the conservative turn toward Christian Democracy seemed everything else but a miracle. The soothsayers and commentators were obviously afraid that this boy, this bastard, kitted out with metaphorical *Star Wars* power but also real "power" could drag a Germany just coming to terms with its own guilt into a new, even more dreadful guilt. Worse, my stepfather, who was prone to alcoholism and violent rages, was called Helmut, and the "Helmut, Helmut" shouts that accompanied Kohl's as well as Schmidt's appearances struck me in this already somewhat mad look back as not merely political howls but indirect prods in the direction of *his* screwed-up psyche, the shouts of hysterical mobs left me retrospectively outraged. I pursued questions of population growth, studied income statistics, and the irregular rhythm of holidays. I dragged these almanacs around with me, leafed through them, compared them with the dates of my own life, and drew ever newer conclusions that seemed to grow clearer and clearer. When exactly was my mother taken to the clinic for psychosomatics? When exactly did I start school temporarily in Godesberg, when did we flee from Aachen? When did the police come? When was the day of the bloody tennis racket? I began extracting the events of my life from the historic happenings, not the other way around. And it all fit, it fit again and again, because I kept forgetting everything and kept entering new cycles of interpretation. If our house was in flames, the whole world was in flames. If the whole world was in flames, our little house exploded.

29

Under water, in waves of sound, that's how I imagine the beginning of my life, a torrent tossing me into the complications of a working-class couple that disintegrated before my memory became operative. Then careened headfirst into the next trap, which was a real one, with the sprung metal bar that slams shut and the rancid cheese, double-bottomed compartments, pitfalls, smears of nosebleed, and the wild demons of Haribo. On TV Helmut Kohl was spreading out rapidly.

It is stupid to settle on one single cause, and it is equally stupid not to look for causes at all. Of course, there are causes in your childhood, even if I find it hard to define them precisely or ensure they don't cohere into a facile explanation of what happened later.

The developing illness caught up with someone who was already on the run. The unrest and bewilderment of childhood had come back. I'd gone to university at nineteen in order to finally construct my own life, according to my own principles and directives. I wanted to get away, just away from the narrow constraints, and out into the world of the intellect and literature, into broadband learning.

Once, when we were watching Super-8 home movies from the seventies, there was one of my parents and me on holiday in Spain. They separated right after, so I can't have been three years old, and the way my mother dragged me along, not letting me take even a few steps on my own though I obviously *wanted* to, the way she kept picking me up and putting me down, attentive but at the same time showing off and almost abusive in her care, as though I were some kind of toy—flirting with the camera at the same time—horrified me. My cousins picked up on it, too, as we watched those movies at Christmas, and kept telling her to lay off. "Hey," they said, as though they could intervene, "just leave Thomas alone, geez!" I couldn't believe it, I looked over at my silent aunts, embarrassed. So *that's* how it was.

The blast of the first divorce (after gambling excesses and debts, after he'd been threatened by pimps and lost a few teeth) must have triggered total instability, which made a life of regular routine impossible. Trying to escape was part of daily life. The desolation of my mother, who herself had been transplanted from Poland to a foreign and foreign-speaking Germany when she was only seventeen, was passed on to me, the sometimes hysterically spoiled and sometimes neglected only child that I was. Looking for a patch of stability, she headed, thoughtless, into a second marriage, with an alcoholic computer programmer, whose violent tendencies were already evident before the wedding. But yearnings are blind. The bloody scenes multiplied, the cycles of separation became more frenzied; more and more often I took on the unhealthy role of protecting my mother, then comforting her, and finally being her emotional *partner*, until the monster was let back into the family cell only to brutally berserk around in it again. That is how trust in anything like a moment of happiness is destroyed: a charmer who was taken in as "Father" keeps turning into an ogre, the mother becomes an abused child, and in the process, the child unlearns how to communicate and retreats into himself. He comforts and comforts, but also ends up on the floor one day, enduring minutes of the boot. All that in less than four hundred square feet of a coal-stove-heated apartment on the wrong side of the tracks.

"My childhood has the colour of a hematoma." That's what I had one of my *Saturday Night* characters say a few months before the first manic attack. He was a failed DJ named Pecker, who spent his time in the basement cutting back and forth between different musical genres and never getting discovered. I know more or less what I meant

by that, I can see the synesthesia of it, but I can also see
the pathos of someone taking a look back at a childhood
that has for the first time become analyzable. The *colour* of
the *word:* because that word often appeared in the medical reports and the doctor's notes—*hematoma*—probably
in order to record the crimes of the monster my mother
had married for occasional court injunctions and perhaps
later, finally, for divorce proceedings. At first, I didn't know
what the word *hematoma* meant, but I figured it out from
the context, and it gave me quite a new perspective on the
events, an objective, third perspective, that of a doctor I
didn't know, but who used precise and neutral terms, pep-
pered with technical terminology, to describe the life we
were living as a catastrophe. Besides comics, these reports
were my first sustained reading experiences.

Anything positive was poisoned. *Heidi* for instance,
Heidi and the police. Five or six years earlier, when we were
living in Aachen, my stepfather sat down next to me one
evening to watch *Heidi,* a series I loved, just like everybody
else. A few weeks earlier they'd bought a video recorder
and I couldn't believe that you could watch everything
over and over again, even *Heidi.* It was an absolute wonder:
reproducible happiness. I had been more or less neglected
for some time, much to my joy and relief—my biological
father had suddenly been to court to extract me "from
those conditions," and when he lost the case disappeared
again, and my mother had begged me with tears in her
eyes and the document in her hand, "You're staying with
me, aren't you?"—and so I found the attention my stepfather was offering that evening both surprising and disconcerting. Where was my mother? No answer. We sat in the
pitch darkness, with only the TV gushing out garish Tech-
nicolor *Heidi* images, and silently watched one program

after the next. He put his arm around me and was patting me. This closeness was new, and fake, but still, I enjoyed it. I didn't realize that, as so often, he was completely drunk, probably high on his pills, and probably in need of comfort himself. I didn't realize there'd been a ruckus at a party in some dive, where he'd lost it and threatened my mother and the neighbours and maybe even gotten violent. The session lasted quite a while; I could smell his sweetish alcohol breath, which I couldn't yet identify as such. Then the doorbell rang: the police. A huge uproar. They wanted to arrest him, the neighbours were there behind them, there was pushing and shoving and yelling and shouting, my mother in tears in the middle of it all. *That* background noise. And I was on my own again with *Heidi,* who now looked quite different.

It went on and on. The value of every gesture of affection was lost in what came next. Around this time, the two of us fled from Aachen back to Bonn, staying with my grandparents at first and then in the dilapidated apartment below, where we lived for many more years—and to which, absurdly and to my horror, my stepfather returned. ("There's a surprise for you at home," my mother said on the way back from my grandparents'—it was Christmas again—"I don't know if you'll be happy about it.") And so this escape, too, lost its value and its purpose. It seemed impossible to escape from anything. The inevitable always returned, and now this guy was back in the house, inexorable, impossible to get rid of, and he soon turned back into his usual disgusting self, lying drunk on the couch and flipping cigarette butts onto the floor, one after the other, to humiliate my mother, who picked them up, one after the other, in tears—and I was supposed to be happy? Over the next few years, it was me and not him who had to fetch two buckets of coal from the basement every day, scared stiff at the various body parts buried under the piles of coal, straight out of the trash TV that ran constantly upstairs, scared stiff at the murderers lurking in the cellar, straight out of the *Express* I had to steal from the newspaper box every morning, scared stiff at the curved volute at the bottom of the banister that, from a certain angle, always resembled the skull of a demon peering around the corner, his sweaty hair stuck to a pallid forehead. Only when I read Stephen King's *It* a year later was I freed from these fears. When horror is fictionalized, it liberates.

"We were not well then," my mother said later. She probably meant the sleeping tablets that both of them consumed in vast quantities: *Lexotanil.* Another un-understood word from my childhood.

30

Half man! Keep moving. I stayed on the top of the wave that was swallowing me whole. Copied hundreds of flyers with William Blake poems and *Spex* interviews that I distributed in Charlottenburg, handed Diedrich Diederichsen, who was hurrying by, an interview I'd oddly enough done with him. Diederichsen was interested at first, and then took off quickly when he recognized the crazy man as a crazy man. Rushed on through the different neighbourhoods, into the parties, accosted people I didn't know, thinking I'd met them online, and even when they said they didn't know me, I insisted that it was precisely in how they said this that I knew who they were—a mad comedy of errors was under way, but the comedy part was pretty limited.

Come on out! I kitted out the foyer of an apartment house with felt-tip scribbled papers, which caused my first encounter with the police, since my paranoid greetings had

been perceived as threats. At a meeting of a group of litera-
ti I kept firing off unfiltered jokes, went on to the Paris Bar
with them, where I chatted some cultural affairs journalist
into a fit of laughter, and later started crying in a taxi with
a graphic artist. She looked shocked as she handed me her
share of the taxi fare and got out. At the university computer centre, I glimpsed an exchange student's email address.
and zipped off a message to her that was actually meant
for someone else, which she thought was incredibly funny,
and during a smoke break outside, I could sense she was
interested in more than trading phone numbers. But that's
not where I was at. Instead, I drifted off into near-sacred
realms, surfing away into metaphysics, in search of the
next clue in the swelled-up and gruesome summer puzzle.
I fled Dahlem, burst into the S-Bahn, stomped through the
compartments, talked nonsense, and kept handing out my
flyers with the copied *Spex* interviews, proverbs and Novalis quotes. Later, at some happy hour, a guy who'd observed
me on one of these excursions, described me as a strange
bird to his girlfriend; "Look, Lara, there's that strange bird
I told you about." I thought that was great or open-minded,
or whatever, and I told Andreas he absolutely needed to
meet this person who'd described me as a strange bird. The
two of them looked at each other in silence, and Andreas
turned to me, and asked, "Why?" When I didn't answer,
he repeated the question, shrugging his shoulders: "Why?"
He was right. I didn't know why. A little question like that
can briefly put the ground back under your feet. The group
dispersed.

Dolphins came leaping out of my mouth, and colourless,
green ideas slept furiously. Magda and I attended a reading
held by the pop culture quintet Tristesse Royale; I brought
along Theodor Adorno's *Minima Moralia: Reflections from*

Damaged Life and my *Saturday Night* manuscript, and so was specially armed. I sat at a café table with Magda, smoking a cigarette and ashing it into the Adorno book with the odd explanation that I was in the process of being burned alive, here and now. I kept translating what the pop culture guys onstage were saying into messages concealed below the surface racket. Magda was completely stymied and fell silent. People kept looking over at us, unsettled. When the reading ended, I fell upon the group of writers standing there together, kept yelling out Alexander von Schönburg's last name since it struck me as so amazingly telling, hit on Christian Kracht, who gave me a hug when he heard my name and then stepped back in a fright and said, "You're an asshole." I liked that, it struck me as Krachtian, and mouthing off loudly I offered him my manuscript, which he didn't want. I liked that too. I laughed and abruptly tossed the manuscript onto a café table and left.

Always there for me, always trying to contain me, calm me down, bring me back, were my friends. And it did actually help to have one of those people I knew and trusted next to me. Their questions would qualify some of my ideas and minimize their more drastic aspects through repetition; they would end up sounding stale, no longer needing to be brashly pushed out, at least not in the next five minutes. Friends also shielded me from the rest of the world. I could temporarily unburden myself without creating a social scandal. For a short time, it was good.

Once, I was at a playground with Lukas, a party going on behind us, where I'd had a few outbursts. Lukas had pushed a bottle of beer at me and lured me to the dark playground where we were now sitting on two swings, downing our beer just like in *The Truman Show*. His glasses made his intelligent, gentle eyes look smaller and his pupils were lit up in duplicate by the moonlight. The rocking horses on their steel springs stood still and listened, the sand scrunched under our shoes. A swell of words burst out of me and I started sounding off about always getting screwed, how everything was shit, that I didn't know how I was supposed to live with it all. But it was more despair than anger, and my tirades were soon accompanied by sobbing. "How are you supposed to live if everything is already a huge fraud, if you're always being cheated, and ratted on and sold out?" I was in tears. Lukas didn't know what to say—it was too late to contradict the paranoia—and when he laid his hand on my back to comfort me, his eyes also filled with tears, although he tried to smile.

31

And so the nights, the days, and the weeks blazed away. I stole, I raged, I yelled. The outward image I presented was frightening and bizarre: a person who could get enthusiastic about all kinds of things but who was also somewhat introverted, who suddenly flared into a thousand idiocies, tossing around nonsensical hypotheses, storming from one strangeness into the next, internally sealed off, no longer accessible, though externally all the more present. Outwardly, it was a psycho-carnival, inwardly paranoia about the past and semantic madness were raging furiously. I was a true human experiment, the long-awaited messiah who had turned out to be a perfectly normal person and was therefore killing off all religions, and all teleologies. Through my normality, we were moving into a new, rationally driven paradise that reconciled myth and enlightenment, and whose possibilities and meaning were being fought over daily, with real weapons and casualties on all sides. It was obvious: Nietzsche hadn't been able to write God to death, but in my ignorance I had simply lived him to death.

32

This view of the world has come up more or less identically in each of the three manic attacks I have endured, and so I want to sketch it out here. I already described it from the inside in the short story "Dinosaurs in Egypt," but there I used a simulated, artistically fictionalized maniacal frenzy, along with the manic-depressive's addiction and other incomprehensible examples. Here, however, I would like to explain.

I assumed there was a secret world history, a secret record dating from the earliest beginnings, a truth that was so universal and so unspeakable it couldn't be revealed to me; I had to figure it out myself, I had to make that leap of consciousness on my own. When exactly this had happened, no one could possibly know, but my idea was that over the centuries hopes for a messiah, quite similar to the Jewish idea, had developed, but were not limited to any one religion or culture. That a messiah would come, around the turn of the millennium, had been whispered and passed on in metaphorical language. This secret eschatology, I imagined, had for centuries suffused all texts, songs, and images in ambiguous ways, exactly as I had recently seen happening online. It was *exactly* this form of expression since it permeated all communication, from the simple purchase of cigarettes at a kiosk to Goethe's *Faust, Part II*, which was why I could now find references to this dark, abstruse complex in texts, films, and images from before I was born. Hopes for a messiah had always existed, but these whisperings, this *one-will-come* that mothers had been singing to their children had spread around the entire world much more tenaciously than earlier prophesies. Very slowly a hysteria had developed, whose true dimensions would only become visible through some wild time lapse. The process was so slow that people no longer knew which hysteria was lodged in the central core of all things.

A race toward the future had been held and of course it was Hitler who, like Stalin, had wanted to construct a new world to prepare for and pre-empt this coming, in order to control all eventualities within the frame of the "Thousand-Year Reich" and at the same time dispel any further hopes for a messiah. Hitler had in the end believed that he was me—that was my manic view. The fact that he thereby focused the world's attention on this cerebral and rhapsodic spot called Germany was both his achievement and his downfall. Instead of killing off the hopes for a messiah, he'd further stoked them. His preposterous delusion had had a further consequence: the most monstrous human crime ever committed had been carried out in my name, before I was even born.

It is pretty clear that the role of such a perfidious messiah is not simple. Suddenly everything is about you, and in order not to put an end to it all with a quick slash of a sacrificial knife (which I sensed would envelop the world in unbelievable darkness: total war and apocalypse, Sodom and Gomorrah), you devote yourself to pop culture. Pop celebrates the moment and makes the effects of paranoia seem less painful. I was glued to MTV, I dissected the radioactively beaming faces of the moderators and accorded great interest to the most trivial tune. But my sense of taste was not completely gone. I still found certain products incredibly irritating, for instance a hit titled "Blue" about a man who is blue, and lives in his blue room, and sings, *I'm blue da ba dee da ba da*, a simplification that was cashing in on my own situation through sheer mockery. In other songs such as Moby's "Why Does My Heart Feel So Bad," I discovered a melancholic pathos that corresponded to my own hopeless condition and moved me to tears. I dug up old CDs, tossed them into the CD player, and listened to them again. Everything had a secret meaning. CDs and books were spread all over the floor. Films and film clips ran on TV. Messages were coming in from all over the place. My room was falling into disrepair.

33

What would the end of the millennium bring? The date alone made it a massive change, one supported by Jesus analogies: *Two thousand zero-zero, party over, oops, out of time,* as Prince expressed it. I was overcome with the feeling that I was being catapulted out of time before it was time. Did everyone who'd understood this worldwide accident and grasped it in its madness really have to flip out like this, and was I simply the last one in line? Is that why Werner Schwab had drunk himself to death? And Sarah Kane killed herself in King's College Hospital? Was that why Rainald Goetz, who was actually a promising doctor, cut open his forehead, lost it completely, and as a controlling icon of the cultural scene never really found his way back? Had Thomas Pynchon really referred to my coming in *V.?* Pynchon—he'd done a much better disappearing act, with his hallucinogenic and clear-sighted dystopias. And yes, of course, he adopted more optimistic tones in *Vineland*, as a lecturer in Tübingen had assured me with a wink two years earlier—of course, because the great monster that had so long been on the horizon (how long exactly?) had turned out to be a little apprentice poet and not, as feared, an insensate dictator or megalomaniac fomenter of religions. Humanity could therefore not be all bad.

We are all bait, baby! is what I kept hearing from all sides. Why had 1982 been so catastrophic? I'd managed to tuck away all the trauma without a whimper! I hiked over to the Literary Colloquium, talked to Bret Easton Ellis after a reading and tried to extract some information from him. I ended up confessing how hard it was to bear the burden of *American Psycho* all alone. Capitalism has a soul, I told the head of the Literary Colloquium over the phone, and he agreed with me.

When I ran out of money, I just invaded stores and openly stole all the CDs and books that had long been my right since they were all intended for me, and were quite simply all about me, and in any case, ever since my time in Austin in 1996, I had contaminated and influenced them all. Everybody had plagiarized me, but in a kind of homage. Because not only had my recent texts been copied by the millions and translated across the web, but the experimental, English-language short stories, theoretically accessible to any citizen of the world, that I'd written in a creative writing course taught by the Pakistani American writer Zulfikar Ghose (and that presaged my current thrown-ness in spooky ways—what clairvoyance!), those texts, too, had been copied and distributed, returning to Germany via the rapid data autobahn, spreading on from there into the world, and becoming a secret canon that everyone referred to. I even listened to every detail of the Fantastic Four's aptly titled 4:99 album, where every line held an allusion and every rhyme a greeting. Trent Reznor stepped out of his misanthropic isolation and in *The Fragile* intimated the darkness lying ahead of me because he'd already lived through it all for me. I couldn't stop letting his music throb into me, fuelling it with beer, fascinated and lost in this new cosmos closing around me. I became more and more hysterical as the end of the millennium approached.

In a hectic need for action, I travelled to Bonn to see if I could find some answers there. In the interim, the Rhine, which in contrast to the laughable Spree, was a real river, calmed me down. My mother had half a nervous breakdown when I explained that the pop singer Patrick Lindner actually meant me when he mentioned his adopted son on a talk show. The people on TV seemed to have changed: they had a stoned glow in their eyes; they were all on some kind of drugs, or they were secretly happy that the prophecies were about to come true, and a new paradise was within sight. You could read it in their love-drugged eyes.

Oh yes, love, love and sex. I was finding love everywhere, but its counterweight and camouflage, hatred, was there too, ensuring I wouldn't suffocate in all the love. An internal inversion took place, and I destroyed what I had always loved. The people nearest me became the most distant and the most distant moved close. Old friends and partners suddenly seemed ignoble traitors, and I resorted to projections that also beset me—books, songs, films, articles. Everything I had loved and lived so far was wrong, ran my thinking, and only in a stranger, who admired me from a distance and whose admiration I tremulously returned, could I recognize any form of innocence.

And sex? I felt more and more like a fetish. If everybody knew me and had thought about me, and was still thinking about me, then I must also be playing a role in their relationships and sexual adventures. I suddenly related S&M practices to myself; within the framework of the monumental distortion whose centre I constituted, the most perverse sex games were mere variations on the attempt to come to terms with an abnormal sex drive, with the thousandfold echo of the bodies. And when you hear your name in the moans of the porn flicks, you are, of course, convinced that all the women of the world need to be available whenever you want. But I wasn't allowed; I had become a sort of holy man. Later, that changed.

AIDS, on the other hand, was an invention, the disease did not exist. It was a creation of the media designed to protect the world from some effect. But what effect? And what would be the result? Would the supposed AIDS victims finally show up again at the turn of the millennium?

Lukas dismantled my modem before Christmas so that I couldn't pump any more nonsense into the internet, and he persuaded me to go back to the psych ward. But I took off after a short stay—a pattern that would repeat itself over the years. The clock was ticking faster and faster, it was almost New Year's Eve. I went to internet cafés and posted new stuff online, on all kinds of forums, in order to measure the relationship between intervals, effects, and reactions. I could hardly read normal news anymore, and whenever I did, it triggered misinterpretations and defiance. It was all a big spectacle, a megalomaniac drama, that was quite empty, with only me, and therefore nothing, at the centre of the media circus. Because what did people actually know about me? I tried to ignore all that, as I had for decades. But it was no longer possible.

34

We celebrated New Year's Eve together. Sitting there with the others, I didn't have much to say and misunderstood most of what they said. The pressure in my head was enormous. Someone had the idea of ringing Ben Becker's doorbell, a floor down, and that's what we did. Very fleshy, very cool, and very hammered, he hung there in the door frame and muttered something. I don't remember anything else, except that I got lost somewhere on the way to a party in the Quietest Club in the World, where Aljoscha, whom I barely knew, was the DJ—that much I remember. And that the clouds of smoke came together in a wall of fog over Berlin-Mitte, it all smelled singed and I traipsed through it, with nowhere to go, its dark whiteness before my eyes. And that I heard about Yeltsin's resignation and thought, now that I'm here he's resigning because he knows America's finally the winner. Let him guzzle vodka. That's what I was doing.

35

An almost tragic bonus of the illness in my case was that there suddenly seemed to be explanations: for how stubborn people were, their inhibitions, the ambiguities, the insults. My relations with others had been so complicated before, and my personality basically so lonesome, that these new and sick insights finally made clear what had gone wrong. No wonder people hadn't been able to have normal relationships with me. And all those horrors in my childhood, the sudden moves, the silences—I could now see clearly why everything was so complicated and so catastrophic: because of the accident of the world! In my non-psychotic moments this explanation subsided, and things were just as twisted and lonesome as before, no, they were more twisted and more lonesome. It was just that now a solid psychic illness had joined the entire baleful complex.

36

The breakdown came at the end of January. I'd moved to Prenzlauer Berg in the meantime (how I did that Robben & Wientjes may know) and was living in a small, comfortable one-room apartment, where I grew calmer. My usual thoughts resumed, and with them the realization that all my assumptions of the past months had been wrong, and not only wrong—no, completely crazy. This realization arrived bit by bit. First, I noticed that some of my ideas about the world couldn't possibly be right, and that the entire megalomaniac counterhistory I'd woven about myself didn't withstand examination under less frantic conditions. Over two or three days, my paranoia collapsed like cold, wet foam. I grew clearer. Neurons stopped overheating and started shutting off. The countless messages once accumulating in my head grew scant. My brain powered down, my mind darkened and was suddenly corroded by an all-encompassing sorrow. What was happening?

When you are confronted with such a condition for the first time—but why "confronted" since the condition doesn't actually face you, it overruns your entire person—so when you are first *befallen* by such a condition, you are devastated, you don't know how to deal with it. The situation is completely new, a horrendous novelty, and there is no category into which you can slot what you are experiencing. What is this? Is this a depression? Why is it so intense, so stark, and so painful? The clearer things become, the darker the patient's world, and even worse, your reactivated consciousness injects you with unspeakable shame, which drags you down even more, hour by hour.

37

It is hard to imagine a life that is more full of shame than that of a manic-depressive. The reason is that such a person lives three different lives, lives that are separate, make war on each other, and shame each other: the life of the depressive, the life of the manic, and the life of the temporarily recovered patient. This patient does not have access to what the other two did or did not do, or what they thought. As the temporarily recovered patient (temporary, because the disorder is permanent and you can only hope that outbreaks remain infrequent), you wander around in tatters, surprised at the battlefield you've left behind you. You can't change anything even though the manic who rampaged there and the ailing depressive are two versions of your self (but who is that?) that can be connected by memory, but hardly by identity. Still, there's no doubt: it was you. You are the one responsible for all the actions, all the disasters, and all the absurdities, you were the excesses, the miscalculations, the obsessions and the meaningless verbiage, the exclusion orders and the suicide attempts, the embarrassments, the rampages, the breakdown. You were the ruffian, and then you were the corpse. And now you are the one with the bipolar disorder, and you are alienated, by definition.

In this constellation, the manic is the noisiest, and the shame is due to his idiotic actions. What an asshole! What a fool. Tearing around the city, on the lookout for the next stupid activity, yet another embarrassing performance heckling someone, yet another side mirror torn off a car, caught in a constant chatter that is always all about you, always being addressed and defamed by things that have nothing and everything to do with you. With neurons fired up and misinterpreting every single aspect of the world, identifying with sex toys, film plots, and historic battles. As a manic with schizoid tendencies you suffocate in your battle against the crazy system that is you, that began with an erroneous feeling, a mistaken interpretation, which triggered two untrue conclusions as well as three mad assumptions, all of which developed a dynamics that can overturn the world in a matter of minutes. Then you take off, in my case for many months, and dissolve in a tangle of time and madness. At the end of it all your reputation and life are in ruins.

It's different for the depressive. You're sprawled out on shards of glass, hardly daring to move. In fact, you can't move. After all your faculties shut down, every day is a void, and you vegetate in a struggle against suicide, which for a depressive is actually not that easy because you're far too paralyzed to make an exit. Every errand is a massive undertaking, every glance a humiliation. The memory of the manic period is torture. And realism plays no part. The mania has simply turned into its opposite. Black is as black as it can never be. But this phase passes eventually; it just lasts about twice as long as the manic phase.

And now, the temporarily healthy person stands there, amid overturned chairs. You cannot trust yourself to do anything, you're performing a balancing act, and you can only pray that the medication will work. The temporarily healthy person—I already wrote about this—has someone inside they cannot rely on; no, you have many of them inside you, a whole army of uncertain recruits and eternal deserters. And when you take an honest look at yourself, open and direct, in the smeared and tarnished mirror, then your life, the way you imagined it, wasted, screwed-up, gone. And any other possibility is a long way off.

If you are manic-depressive, your life no longer has continuity. Whatever there was as a more or less coherent history falls apart as you look back on disconnected bits and pieces. The illness has shot your past to pieces, and presents an even more dire threat for your future. Every manic episode makes your life as you once knew it even less possible. The person you thought you were and you thought you knew no longer has a solid foundation. You can no longer be sure of your self.

And you no longer know who you were. You don't recognize your actions although you can remember them. During a manic short-circuit, some idea that might otherwise briefly flare up and be immediately suppressed, turns into an action. Every person probably has a certain abyss inside them, that they occasionally acknowledge with a glance; a manic attack, however, is a full-fledged tour of this abyss, and whatever you knew about yourself for years becomes invalid, in the briefest span of time. And afterward you don't just start at zero again, no, you slide down into the deepest minus-zone where nothing connects to you in any reliable way.

Who has the strength to construct anything new from there?

38

I sit there, I am an object. I no longer belong to the class of humans but have joined the inanimate: objects, things, items: soulless and dead. The people around me are nothing but inanimate objects either, though I know better. Their words, if there are any, hardly reach me. I know this is not how things are, but that is how I feel them. I am made of wood, or steel, or plastic, my veins are cables. I feel nothing but grief. The universe in which I sit is minuscule and motionlessly cold. The ventilation system is humming like in a David Lynch film, an unfeeling, empty background buzz. I go to the toilet, the bathroom fan kicks in and heralds nothing. I keep hearing it, an obsessively mocking resonance of nothing. I never used to hear it. It used to be on the other side. Now I am with it.

I am twenty-four years old, but time has gotten lost and

me with it. Time is either absent, a frightening vacuum where nothing happens, or it is a brittle fabric that closes in on me and slowly benumbs me. The apartment is hostile and silent. I didn't want to come here. How did I get here? The apartment is a hostile refuge that I, as a boneless parasite, can hardly leave, because if I do I'll have to go out into the sunshine that blinds me, and I'll have to be around people, that is if I even recognize them as living beings, in another, unreachable world, behind glass, apparently in other dimensions, of a completely different kind and constitution. I know from a distance what it's like to be them. Today, that is quite impossible.

I am profoundly ashamed. If I let myself go, I can completely immerse myself in the shame. And I have to let myself go, because I can't defend myself. I disappear into this shame hourly. Moments come sloshing up, morbid strings of thought, mistaken thoughts, mistaken systems. But especially incidents, situations, and actions spiked with abnormalities and absurdities. I was all that? Flashbacks, eyes shut, waves of shame. I can't distance myself from it, I can't call my own behaviour "bizarre" or "absurd," I can't objectify it or keep it at bay, that's how weak I am. I have to push it aside for a second, just long enough to get up and look in the fridge, which is empty. There's a light in there, related in its pallid artificiality to the bathroom fan. Everything is real, really dead.

I sit there. I am nothing. Something is sitting there and is no longer.

39

Spring arrived, the first part of the *Big Brother* series had been running for awhile. I could remember exactly—it had only been a few weeks—experiencing the shrill *Big Brother* ads in the TV magazines as a personal insult, a mockery aimed at me. Now *Big Brother* was on the air, an example of the paltry media productions that were the rule, a thin plot, driven by even thinner voyeurism. Still, this mix was just tepid enough for me to watch it every now and then and briefly forget who and how I was. I was too wrecked to take in novels or movies. Then I would fall asleep, as soon as I could, and wake up hating the sun that shone straight in my face in the morning because I couldn't get it together to install curtains or move the bed away from the window. To sleep forever, please, and not to dream. Not a second made any sense, not even in my imagination.

I travelled to Bonn and stayed there a few days. Konrad and Malte thought *Big Brother* was a cool parody and wanted to go to Cologne to help celebrate Zlatko Trpkovski's departure. I went along because I didn't know what else to do with myself. I had nothing to say during the trip. I admired Konrad and Malte for how normal they were, their jokes, their sarcasm, I was familiar with the somewhat dishonest attitude of ironically undertaking a low-end activity but really loving it deep down. I couldn't access that myself though. I just went along, passive, stood in the dark among a group of people, we took off somewhere, saw nothing, and drove back. The others had a good time, I had nothing. That was no longer a lump in my throat, it was an occlusion.

My mother cooked for me and turned out to be a heroine of affection and patience, having undergone many depressions herself. But it didn't help.

I availed myself of various psychotropic drugs that she, unreasonably, had decided not to take. They were in a little vial, a whole bunch, especially Tavor. I didn't ask for any information, I just thought, that'll be enough.

40

I get in the train back to Berlin, and I know as I watch my mother waving outside that I will unfortunately never see her again. We are both in tears, though neither of us wants to recognize this. Our faces are distorted in pain. The tears keep coming but are discreetly brushed away. Why hide it, I think, why so secretive? As the train starts moving, as in a film—but it's not a film, it is the saddest reality ever—a suffocated scream rises between us. I can't help but imagine myself dead. This is truly the last goodbye, I'm not the one who decided, something else decided for me: this life is no longer worth living. I don't know if she knows, but I reckon she knows and is pushing it aside. I am so sorry, and I cry more over her than over myself, which I find both fake and pretentious. But why keep on dissecting the pain, it is everywhere.

Back in Berlin, the apartment feels quiet and dry. Time is torture. I no longer know what to do with anything, with the songs, the books, the movies. My always rather precarious relationship with people is completely finished. When I try to apologize, my friends still tell me I don't need to apologize. They understand and are glad the nightmare is over. For me it has only just begun. They've grown through all of this; I am wasting away.

The days pass in agony. Depression is not a lack of feeling, which is what I had imagined, it is a constant humiliation, a sharp, steady pain, instability, and grief. I shut my eyes and think, this can't be true. I open my eyes and nothing has changed. I shut my eyes, I open my eyes. Then I go to bed, but I can't fall asleep. Then I do fall asleep, and sigh when I wake up.

I put the pills in the kitchen cupboard, next to the plates. The cupboard looks so orderly; who lives here? A tidy female student? Why is this apartment so clean and new, but small? There's the old kitchen table. I never sit there. To try it out I sit down at it. Nothing. I sit down at the computer. Nothing. I lie down, I stand, I walk. My accompanying thoughts are limited to exactly the same: I lie down, I stand, I walk. Even the question about where my thoughts have gone can no longer be asked. There is absolutely nothing left.

Another day. And another one. No improvement.

Another one. I can't keep on.

Another week. Another day.

It's over.

41

I remember the horror on Lukas's face when he opened the door and saw me lying there on the couch, unconscious. Did he wake me up? I remember his wide-open eyes behind the glasses, the terror in them. He'd tried to reach me, and when he couldn't he imagined the worst. I'd taken the pills, big, loaf-shaped boats and small blue coins. I'd taken all of them, about a hundred and fifty, and lain down. Lukas had rung the bell, then knocked, and then hammered on the door. Somehow he got into the apartment. Did he have a key? Probably. He'd become responsible for me, he was on my side. There was always someone on my side, but these friendships usually did not survive the effort they demanded; all the work wore them out.

We drove off. On the way to the clinic I felt clear in the head, and was surprisingly present. But weeks later, Lukas pointed to a completely sedated, slobbering, trembling specimen in the closed ward and said, "That's about what you looked like. Yeah, it's tough, but that was more or less the picture."

This time, my stay in the clinic was not voluntary. I had no will left anyway.

42

They put me in the same dark, stone-age-like ward as they had months earlier, but this time the perspective had changed radically. What was once a way station in my pseudo-comic carnivalesque and hectic quest had turned into a dim, ground-floor prison with barred windows, where time seemed just as confined as the inmates. But I had no complaints, because as I said, I had become a person without a will. I let whatever had to be done be done; I checked off food orders on a yellow sheet of paper for delivery in two days' time, was a little surprised I would apparently still be alive in two days' time and was also surprised that the foods I had checked off actually appeared on the table two days later. The future could apparently be checked off.

My memories range from foggy to nil. The former patients, the ones I had known, were gone, Annoying Olaf and Herr Direktor had been replaced by other faces. Alcoholics and depressives played skat together, and I watched though I didn't understand the game. People used the coffee machine like a trough in the morning, me included. And while just months ago I'd lectured a suicidal conscientious objector about his cowardice, I had now become like him, silent, never smiling, huddled into myself, and mercilessly inaccessible. I remember comforting Magda, who was in tears beside me, and awkwardly putting my arm around her. I had cried over her at first, secretly, because something had been developing between us again—a growing interest on her part, a manic infatuation on mine—but then things had overwhelmed her, understandably, and when I came to she was in a new relationship. Now she was in tears beside me, and I hugged her in her helplessness, but she was actually crying over mine. Maybe I briefly felt human again.

Apart from that moment, the numb lack of feeling I had long been promised now set in. With the exception of one nighttime incident when I sat down on a chair in the corridor and burst into silent but convulsive tears, which made a nurse come over and try to console me, I turned to stone inside, I'm tempted to say I *finally* turned to stone inside. I had been miserable for too long; now the condition petrified and no longer triggered sharp pain. The anti-depressants and the prophylactics were having an effect too. The grief was there, but shock-frozen, deep-iced. The days were run by others, their structure, the hours of therapy, the meals and bedtimes. They kept me doing a few things, handicrafts or painting, even if I couldn't take it seriously. But then I painted the same faces I'd painted in my youth, wrinkled, frustrated comic faces, craggy characters that attracted the attention of my co-painters, as they always had, even outside. Earlier, I'd viewed them as arabesques of a certain world view and they'd come together in a work of art driven by my youthful arrogance, but now they were just sick, ridiculous pictures that seemed to be parodies of my earlier skills. My roommate was feeling much the same as he used watercolours to create a naively sinister image of a head that was supposed to have something terrifying about it, but didn't.

"What is it you're trying to say?"

"That's me."

"Why is that you?"

"A monster. I'm a monster."

I never found out what he'd done. With his bulletproof glasses, the long drinker's nose he'd inherited from his ancient mother who visited him every day, and his sadly muttering moustache, I figured he hadn't done much. He had become a monster in his own eyes, and maybe that was worse than any misdemeanour he had actually committed.

The abnormal was normal, and my tired gaze grew even wearier from all the lunacy. I let them have their way with me. I was so spineless I even allowed myself to be used as a specimen for medical students. Probably deep down inside I had some objection, but I couldn't dredge up this indignation or activate it, let alone express it. I just went along. I probably thought that if I didn't really have a use anymore, I might as well function as an anonymous example for the next generation. So I was brought into a wood-panelled seminar room and displayed as a "typical example of an endogenous depression, part of a manic-depressive illness with schizoaffective aspects." I looked at the students' faces, they seemed pretty clueless themselves. A few months ago I was partying and hanging out with you, I thought, and now I'm on the other side. How did that happen! I felt a kind of politeness, some discretion in how they looked at me. I was only twenty-four years old, dammit, and they were maybe two years younger. But I was so much older and heavier and at the same time, more astonished to be in the underbelly of this counterworld, where lives were destroyed in an instant.

The professor, who was also a doctor in the closed psych ward, said a few words that did not put me down. I could imagine what she said before I arrived or once I left: a brief medical history, bio, psychiatric diagnosis, and please note the expressionless face, the slumped posture, the hanging shoulders, the obvious apathy. *Just a few weeks ago, this person was whirling up and down the corridor like a dervish*, is what she probably told them. *I saw him myself. And now, as you can see—a classic case.*

I was briefly ashamed, and then I was dismissed, I'd literally been exhibited and hadn't had a thing to say about it. It was okay, it was dreadful; it didn't matter. Back to the ward, back to jam, pills, and cigarette butts.

Days like frosted glass, weeks like labyrinths. You trot along with the others, moving from here to there, checking off the silly therapies, waiting for food, killing time smoking. It's a novelty to be one of the real sickos. It's a novelty not to understand yourself at all, to be so cut off, so relieved of all functions, exempt from all responsibilities, to have just ended up somewhere. No one is or has ever been master in their own house. The lack of understanding of your own existence is universal. I was in shock from the madness that had struck my life, from the destruction it unleashed, the devastation. I didn't know that much worse was yet to come, I had no idea how over the next ten years the illness would viciously continue to rage and ravage and ransack. The first great loss had occurred, *the first cut is the deepest*. The biggest shock was that I had lost my self. The I, theoretically a construct but in practice quite a reliable guide, was gone, demolished, rendered nil. And because I was no longer a person, I couldn't see any time, any future before me, nor any chance of climbing back out of this pit.

43

It wasn't patience that helped me survive, it was dumb, benumbed perseverance, a blurry existence under neon lights: the respiratory system just keeps working. The fear of the pain of dying allows postponement. The thousandth cigarette helps you get through the next five minutes of the abyss. And at some point your gaze begins to reawaken, register things, split off from the internal void. Every time another patient flips out it is a welcome change, and the occasional absurdity once again registers as being absurd. That's when you also start to sense the danger. Nobody feels safe, because who knows what just set off the other patient: what demons? what perverse moods? You don't know their histories, and everybody lies. The safe space is a powder keg. On the other hand, that usually doesn't matter. In this ward, in these corridors, you're basically dead, cut off from life outside, from oxygen, held behind glass or wood, really lifeless, no longer breathing, dead. And yet, weeks later, your heart timidly starts to beat again.

No matter how rough things are, when you're in a psych ward at some point you start struggling to get out. The first step toward this goal, which you share with the doctors and the nurses, are leaves. I was allowed a leave to go buy cigarettes, an enormous step in the direction of autonomy. The Charité campus was like a garish light installation I stepped into, disconcerted by so much life round about me, so much meaning. Everyone knew where they belonged, what they were supposed to do, where they were going. I stood there in dismay at having no such scenario, knowing nothing, unsure how to take the first step. Still, by the time I was on my fourth or fifth leave, I stopped in at the small campus bookstore and even bought a book by Robert Gernhardt, whose work I'd actually loved and which I then read in sadness. I couldn't share in his humour although I understood it. It didn't elicit a single chuckle, which made me even sadder. (In Bonn, my mother later bought me a book by Christian Kracht, entitled *Der gelbe Bleistift. Reportagen* (The Yellow Pencil. Reports). She'd let me choose, and with a gloomy look on my face, I reached for the nearest item. On the way home from the bookstore, she asked me if I would like the book, and I said yes. I was the little boy again whose interests nobody understood, but who was observed, with benevolence, from outside, from above. The book ended up not speaking to me, not at all, and I don't even think that had to do with me.)

First there were the leaves, nervous and tentative, and weeks later, a night spent at home. The hostile apartment was suddenly a retreat from the terrors of the closed ward. This is one of the perverse effects of psychiatry: you are so stressed and under attack, so ravaged by boredom that the un-places you came from and that you staggered into like a zombie, become more livable again. Because in the psych ward things are a few degrees more horrible than on the outside. I started reading online again, then a few lines here and there in my old books. Every now and then a sentence would cause a distant resonance, and I enjoyed the warm reading light on my writing desk that spread a soft, unclinical twilight glow into my room. I started going out with friends again, to a bar or the movies, saw *Being John Malkovich* for instance, a film I was able to discuss briefly with an intern; I was even able to tell her I'd liked it. That was already a big step forward. My condition improved, without my realizing it. Doctors can identify such developments before the patients do.

While I was watching *Being John Malkovich*, however, the fire department sawed through my window. I'd forgotten a date with Magda and she'd panicked. Was I lying there in my room, dead? The comment from one of the firemen is worth repeating; after he found the apartment empty and after he listened to Magda's explanations, he gestured disparagingly and said, "We're not in the business of making cartoons." It's not that the line is really funny, but when I heard it I had to grin, for the first time in a long time. Still, it took weeks for me to find the strength to sweep up the last shards of glass.

44

"I've read your mother's documents. Things look quite promising."

My mother's documents. She'd faxed the clinic a pile of university transcripts, full-bodied letters of praise from Tübingen and Austin. And that would continue: my mother's faxes in times of crisis, totally bizarre, with her underlinings and handwritten comments. But these testimonies from afar had apparently had some effect on the beautiful doctor, who wore her hair drawn back tightly.

"We'll get you back into shape," she said drily.

I said nothing, but I thought, no.

"Yes, we will," she said, "we'll sort things out," though I hadn't responded.

Later on, I met with a psychologist who used a stone-age computer to measure my reaction times and ability to think logically. After the first few questions, he smiled: "I guess this is about finding out how far above average you are."

Such things still flattered my never-quite-extinguished vanity, but I also thought, no. It's not a question of being above some kind of average. It's only about surviving, regardless of the clichés.

45

No matter how rough things are—you still work at getting out. Even, or especially, if you are still determined to commit suicide. Which is why I started lying to the doctors, or rather to think I was lying to them. They, meanwhile, saw an improvement in my mood that I couldn't see, but which I deployed to confirm their positive findings and declare that things were really much better. I lied, without lying.

Why do all this, I thought, every day is still a burden, I just want to get out, out of here, and then when I'm ready,

I can make my real exit, the way I want to, not determined by someone else, not hectically between two appointments or while stepping out of a tram or just in passing. Ideas like this already imply deliverance. If you're no longer hell-bent on throwing yourself away, you're healing. But for many, this is also one of the most dangerous times: the first fragments of your will are waking up again, the I is slowly feeling its way back, body and soul are gradually stabilizing, but the depression is not completely gone. Many use this window of growing strength to finally act on the decision they made long ago. Before, they were too weak and paralyzed to undertake anything. Now they gather all their budding energy to finally disappear completely.

46

The trendy-looking doctor with the Wayfarer glasses who signs my release forms for the few days separating the psych ward from my new status as an outpatient enters into a "gentleman's agreement" with me. The agreement simply says: *I will not hurt myself.* His part of the deal is to provide my ration of medication. A lonely S-Bahn journey follows with the sun viciously poking at me through the smeared window. Outside, the Legoland of Berlin. At home, silence. Reading, again. Surges of grief, still. The days that go by without a trace. Ping-Pong at the day clinic. First conversations with recovering patients. The tram journeys to and from the clinic, dull, dismal, lost. There is no will, just the duty to keep on, for whatever reason. The idea to write about all this one day. A first visit to a seminar on political philosophy at the Humboldt University, hardly able to take in anything, still fully depressed, no contact with people or ideas, and far removed from my major interests in philosophy of language and consciousness—but still, somehow present. The sun again, that sardonic bitch. People like insects on the Friedrichstrasse, on the way to their beehives, anthills, maggot nests. Me among them, a nothing with no direction. The weight, the train journeys. The senselessness of the internet. I can't get into the internet at all. I spend days at the computer just playing solitaire. Then the idea to run a bookstore. One hour of euphoria about that, and my mother's joy at hearing that now and again I am happy. A meeting with my mentor at the university's funding agency, his talk about "soft skills" that people like me don't need, and his promise of further support. My surprise that, after all, there's some understanding and support available from the bureaucracy. Then again, the hard faces. The months. The song "Alles" (Everything) by the Neubauten. Coldplay's song "Everything's Not Lost." The repeat button on my CD player. The autumn of my first great relief. Shaking it off.

47

Shaking it off. The lowest point of the depression was fading away, the days were acquiring a contour, and so were feelings and thoughts. The sound of the bathroom fan was no longer so intrusive. I was slowly getting better, and night life played an important role.

I was released from the day clinic. At first, I didn't know what to do with myself. University? Absurd. How would that work? I vegetated for awhile, made a first few rounds through the Winsstrasse neighbourhood of Prenzlauer Berg, which was now my home, went to Kaiser's, did some online shopping, and went back to the apartment. The film script a friend wrote and sent me made me happy. So it was possible to actually complete something? My friends were there, were involved, and took me along with them, a personality-less zero. I started going to concerts again, I gingerly set foot in the clubs. Knut was my companion and I was his sidekick, I began to take up more space, with more determination, where I wanted. During the day I returned to my studies, after all. It would be a joke, I thought, if I couldn't finish this program. And that's what I did.

This is when Aljoscha entered my life. I knew who he was from an earlier party at our shared place (a party whose excesses had first driven Lukas and me apart). He'd been standing over against the wall, nodding at me with his penetrating hawk's eyes. He'd come with Knut, who knew him from Cologne. Later in the evening we'd shared our taste for the music of Blumfeld and while the others were already wiped out, Aljosha put on "That's How I Live" and it was clear where we were both coming from.

I remember a concert where I was still a little groggy from the depression, but after downing two beers outside in the evening light with Aljoscha and his girlfriend Bianca, I said, "I've had enough! I'm buying a guitar, I'm going to get myself an electric guitar and I'm going to *slam* my riffs into the strings! Something has to give! I want a guitar!"

"I haven't heard that kind of noise from you, ever. Let's have more of it!" was Aljoscha's answer. And I laughed. I laughed some more, and I knew I was laughing. It felt good.

Overnight the symptoms would abate, and during the day there was regular work. At some point I dropped the medication and instead focused on the healing qualities of beer, books, and music. I started to connect with myself again. I was slowly coming back. The last blurs of the depression dissipated in intoxication. Bianca called the three of us, Knut, Aljoscha, and me, the three musketeers, infantrymen of the night. We fired each other up, and danced in the moment, just having fun. And my connection to Aljoscha grew deeper and deeper, a dark-soul fraternity that we kept resisting by chasing after unfettered moments, any form of fleeting happiness, in art, at the movies, in conversation or in music.

Then I had a girlfriend, who smoked up too much and liked conspiracy theories. I soon found that completely off-putting, a playful variation on the psychosis I had just put behind me but that I could only sense, because I was too young, I knew myself too little, I only had the present and the future on my radar.

September 11 came, and I was glad I wasn't feeling paranoid on the day of those attacks; it was hard to imagine what I might have thought or done. At that point I was working for Forsa, a firm that did public opinion surveys, on the evening of the attacks as well. The reactions of the people on the phones ranged from flustered to panicky. I didn't get yelled at as much as I normally did, and quickly took on the role of therapist, channelling the fears of my fellow creatures just by listening. An older lady asked me if I'd seen the picture of Bin Laden, and then whispered, "He's the anti-Christ, young man, he is truly the anti-Christ. It's time," through the headphones into my ears.

It was time: I had reconstructed myself. The echoes of the explosion still resonated but I was living a life again, biking up and down the Prenzlauer Allee every day, reading, working, doing part-time jobs, partying, loving, fighting. I moved in with my new American girlfriend, shouldered responsibilities, kept writing my stories.

Something had happened, but I didn't see it as an event that might repeat itself. I was a perfectly normal human being, setting up a shared apartment, continuing my studies, looking forward to a lovely life. Only rarely did I talk to my girlfriend or other people about the psychic malfunction, but when I did, I was honest. I also thought the experience made me a tad less arrogant, gave me more empathy for people who had failed or were struggling, and let me take a real interest in anything unique or abnormal, speechless or excluded.

At the end of my studies, after the last oral exam, I sat down in the meadow near the Institute for Comparative Literature with a can of beer in my hand like a quotation. The address of the institute is the rather threatening but lovely "In the black hollow." The sun was shining, it was lunchtime. I thought I could feel Adorno's concept of "reconciliation" that had just been treated theoretically and as pompously as possible in the exam, find its true expression in me. I felt reconciled with everything, I was both subject and object, gently borderless, sitting there with my beer, looking around, completely happy. The trees were friends, the meadow a patch of paradise, the sky sublime and open. I had learned a lot, and it had gone well. The time was ripe for a life. I finished my beer and left the meadow behind, knowing I would never sit there again, and got into the subway, smiling. The chasm that my illness had ripped open in me was now closed.

I wasn't sick. It made sense to drop the medication. It had made me dull and fat, muted things and dumbed them down. The only real remedy I could see in my healing process was time passing. And that was finally on my side again. There'd been a glitch, an intense mishap in the life of a young hothead. Now I could grow up.

2006

I'm at the North Sea, on the island of Sylt. Early evening, the light is failing, actually has already failed, shapeless mist, textured and damp, twilight grey. I'm thinking about Cézanne and how he painted the sea as a vertical wall, and right away I see the sea as an actual vertical wall before me. Am aware that this perception is not real but a rather histrionic wish to see it that way and I give in to the wall. It exudes a calm that embraces me but doesn't soothe me. I think about Ulrich Wildgruber committing suicide on this coast and I want to turn away from the sea that is drawing me nearer and beginning to softly whisper in my ear. But I stay there, and continue to stare at the vertical grey. I withstand all that.

I just trashed the room in which I spent the last two months as a guest at the artists' retreat Syltquelle. I don't know why I trashed it. An emotional catastrophe came rushing through me, a revolt against my fate, which strikes me as unbearable. I have the entire world at my back, all of history. There are no guilty persons, there is only guilt, and it is hanging there over me as an abstraction, a sort of emerging entity that cannot be ascribed to any one person. I threw food around and I tore something up. Once again, my life seems a monumental fraud. I know that feeling, but now I know that my so-called recovery over the past years has been nothing but perfidious self-deception, that has cost many people their lives.

Yes, that's really who I am.

I am the victim of the spirit of the world. I am the one who was flung off the curve as the world turned. It's all exactly as I assumed it was in 1999. How could I have let these years go by without shrieking out against this injustice and offering my privileged position and incredible abilities to the service of humanity. If I hadn't suppressed the insights of 1999, September 11 would not have happened! Just think about that! Just think about that! I stare at the sea again. It's a vertical wall I could run crashing into. The trashed room doesn't matter. Anything goes in the face of this unspeakable injustice. It stinks to high heaven and comes crashing down from the clouds.

2

In turmoil and confusion I trudge back through the sand to Syltquelle. I have to cook something. I just cooked something. What did I cook? Something unique. I have to refine it. Upstairs in my room, I yank open the fridge. It is stuffed chaotically full of too much food. I walked from Westerland to Rantum because I couldn't wait for the bus, because I've run out of patience, with everything. I loaded up my shopping cart in the sad excuse for a grocery store there. Then I paid with some cash I'd been handed. I stuffed the heaps of food into the fridge. These processes were normal and legitimized by bureaucracy. I open the oven door and see the casserole with my meal inside. It looks like a frozen kids' birthday, colourful and effervescent, a mixture of everything, sweet and sour, meat and vegetable, it is incomparable. I turn the oven up again to give the dish a final crusty frosting of heat.

"Is that still edible?" my colleague Nussbaumeder asked in his pragmatic-sarcastic way when he saw the casserole, yesterday, or maybe a few hours ago. I said yes, but was a little perturbed. Maybe I'm in the process of poisoning myself? I keep an eye on the casserole, pace up and down in this luxurious apartment, read the papers and the internet, go over to Nussbaumeder's room to watch *Kulturzeit* on TV with him, and mouth off about the critics. The food is ready, right? Yes. It is unique. It has to cool off.

I carry the casserole down the stairs to expose it to the precious cool sea breezes, which will give the meal a final, very subtle, salty edge. I wait outside. It is completely dark, even the strange restaurant across the way where I drink Averna every day. Then another surge of rage. It's too quiet here, this silence is a total lie! And the meal is all wrong, just stupid; I wanted to do what Nussbaumeder did, a fantastic colleague who likes to cook and share his meals with us in that calm Bavarian way of his. I wanted to invite him, serve up something exceptional, and admittedly also trump him in the culinary arts, triumph even there. A surge of rage courses through my nerves and I briefly see what a fool I am. Then I raise my right foot and let it plunge into the casserole. The brownish mash splatters out in all directions. There need to be traces. I take a few steps in the yard with my foot soaked in meat-mash, demonstrating that I've made a mistake, but was here. It is dark now, but I will see it tomorrow. On the inside, I am furious, tragic, and comic, a hulk of hubris under this Frisian sky. I leave the casserole there, go upstairs, and pour myself a whisky to calm down. It has the opposite effect and I get even more stirred up, more excited, and don't know what to do. The oil painting on the wall is definitely a picture of me. I knew that when I first arrived, at first glance, it was so obvious.

But what I saw as reverence, as a silent offer to live here forever, far from the madness over on the mainland, has now turned into blistering mockery. Besides I don't have a lot of patience for that kind of subtle slimeball flattery from the cultural bureaucrats. I hurl lemons and oranges at the painting. They burst wonderfully, but this doesn't solve anything. I throw more fruit at the ceiling, out the window, nothing happens. I want to play the piano but it's locked. I'm confounded. What am I doing here?

I don't sleep, and leave early the next morning; I flee actually. This hermit-artist residence is not for me, not now. I realize I have not behaved properly. I tell my publisher over the phone they can use the second half of the grant to clean up the room. I'm sorry, I say. I have to get back to Berlin. They won't see me here again.

3

"A true Melle," someone said, grinning, ten years later. During his own Sylt residence he'd shown his wife the stains on the wall and kept thinking "a true Melle." I am obliged to join in the laughter; after all, this is one of the better ways to talk about these things. Humour, even bad jokes, may be the best solution.

4

It happened over New Year's. Before I went to Sylt, I'd been in Erlangen. I was writing for the theatre at this point and was developing a play together with the actors and the director. Developing plays collaboratively was the trend then, nobody knew exactly why. It was soon replaced by a wave of performance art and documentaries.

Theatre was an old passion of mine; as a teenager I'd wanted to become a director, had produced school plays and written short dramas, but then decided to study *something serious* first, namely humanities—which has a certain irony. But at the time it seemed absurd to imagine myself as a creative artist and go directly to one of the schools for dramatic arts. Besides, I only ever wanted to write.

After I developed a play with the up-and-coming Martin Heckmanns that, to everyone's surprise, actually landed in Berlin at the Deutsches Theater in 2004, I received the offer to try something similar in Erlangen. I was still working a day job as a copywriter for an oil company, I'd finished up my studies with an expansive thesis on William T. Vollmann, was labouring over the first versions of *Sickster* and other texts, living half-focused and stable. So much future lay ahead. No thoughts about my illness, I mean, yes, of course I thought about it, but I saw it as something I'd finished with that could now be turned into text, an explosion that hadn't really been understood and had remained unspoken, but that kept resonating over the years. I couldn't imagine that it had just been the prologue to two more, and much more serious, outbreaks. I considered it a one-time occurrence and thought I was out of danger. Doctors refer to this as remission, a phase in which the symptoms subside and even disappear, in order to reappear all the more violently afterward. And the patient's concomitant refusal to see themself as chronically ill and the disease as an integral part of their life is a widespread and all-too-understandable phenomenon. Who wants to drag along such a clubfoot? You just went nuts for a moment, that's all. Dreadful, but it's over. Won't happen again.

5

I was supposed to spend the six weeks of rehearsal in Erlangen, and that's how things looked at first. The actors kept devising improvisations, and developing characters and plot fragments, which I took up and worked on overnight. The scenario I'd set up, against some opposition, was a suicide clinic, the House to the Sun, an institution that was a combination of a government-run human removal system and a wish-fulfillment machine. Each "client" who garnered the privilege to spend their last weeks or months there saw this suicide factory, camouflaged as a clinic or rehabilitation centre, differently: as a beauty farm, a mecca of plastic surgery, an all-encompassing game of strategy, an enormous, last-stop dating site. What was clear to everyone, though, was that the state had calculated the cost of maintaining people who were no longer willing or able to produce and concluded that it was both more humane and cheaper to offer them an option to voluntarily exit life, but with a maximum number of wishes fulfilled. Simulations helped them make their choices. This outline was an enormous fiction machine, a morbid, moody sci-fi dystopia full of hedonism and nihilism, where yearnings still played the biggest role and every figure ended up broken and confused, the way I liked and needed it. I threw myself into the work.

Days were spent in rehearsals, nights in the apartment at the theatre, preceded by a few beers with my colleagues in the bar across the street. Whisky accompanied many a creative nighttime inspiration, and in the mornings I felt destroyed and happy, and arrived at rehearsal with new material. It was crazy. After two weeks, the script was complete, at which point I lost my mind completely.

Theatre, as we know, is a drinking club, even more so at a provincial theatre. You sit around in desolate canteens and wood-panelled bars, downing beer and shots, killing the inescapable and dull togetherness with drivel. This comes with all the psycho-dynamic tensions a dysfunctional family might display, but they play out at high speed. You cling to each other, act out the most intense roles, let conflicts swell and burst open, forge coalitions and develop rankings, confuse fiction and reality, and drink yourself into nirvana. A quiet outsider like me, who is not part of the family, can't help but get caught under the wheels.

At New Year's, during the break in rehearsals which I spent in Berlin, I was already, as a friend put it, "a different person." And my perception had in fact already contracted and narrowed, become somehow two-dimensional. I talked to people as though they were flat, animated surfaces, no longer reaching them. Days and nights of incubation led up to a party at year's end that I no longer remember but that struck me as an immobile tableau, where ideas converged like the proverbial mercury, only sluggishly, in slow motion. I was trapped in the play, as I was trapped in my head.

6

The play took over my reality. I began to see the characters I'd created in people around me and not the reverse, which would have made more sense. The lines I'd written echoed in the conversations I had, other people's comments sounded like new quotes and I gradually came to view the basic idea of the play as a work of genius that brought all our lives, destroyed in late capitalism, to their moment of truth while also foretelling the future. It was with this baggage of ideas that I returned to the theatre.

But what had happened to Erlangen? This ludicrous town that seemed to consist only of a pedestrian zone and a Siemens plant, a town I didn't know and didn't want to know anything more about than what I'd learned from the funny lyrics of the song "What You Need to Know

About Erlangen"—in other words, nothing—this town had changed when I returned on the third of January. It had grown quieter and even more unbearably cozy, and at the same time something was happening—but what? What was going on? I headed out of my theatre apartment and started exploring. A strange scene: full of tension like a closed-down nuclear power plant. I got lost, wandered through a sterile new housing development, and ended up in the same place from where I'd got lost. The system spit me out again at the starting point. A restaurant whose doors stood wide open wasn't open for lunch. The manager shooed me out, making sweeping gestures, though all I wanted was a slice of roast that I was suddenly certain I'd more than earned. Instead, I had one of those baguettes with sun-dried tomatoes that I'd been eating ever since I first arrived, and then found myself back in the pedestrian zone that a couple of the actors had already much maligned, to finally "do lunch" at a restaurant, something I never normally did. I would usually just go to a restaurant, but this time I decided to "do lunch" and had to smile at this semantic shift. I had a beer and focused on the third act of the text which the director wanted to see both loosened up and tightened, an effect I achieved in a moment. The results were acceptable, a heated conversation in fragments that brought the conflicts between the characters to a climax. I started to ponder the names of the characters, consider their etymologies, which I hadn't spent much time on at first but that now seemed to match the figures in a complicated yet almost obscenely precise manner. That was no coincidence, it was not intuition, it was something else: a secret pact between words and objects.

A high school student at a table close by said something funny to his friends. I thought that he was referring to me and I asked whether his little comment was about me. He beamed, no, he hadn't meant me, this was obviously a "mistake" on my part. I briefly thought about this "mistake," and then about my general fear of making mistakes, though I knew that the biggest mistake was probably the constant effort to avoid making mistakes. I decided to take the next opportunity to make a mistake. The pretty waitress who would probably have been described as "luscious" by the sort of person who "does lunch" at a restaurant, was twinkling intensively at me over the glow of the candlelight, expressing something between interest and control, and as the guy who was far too obviously staring and whose gaze was again looking for something that didn't exist, I kept sparking messages back at her. I got up, unfazed, left the place, and headed back to the theatre bar to find nobody there, which struck me as something the others had planned.

Knut, who was visiting me, soon noticed that "something was wrong" again. I was latching on to things and signs; my gaze would wander and flicker all over the place, then catch on some unimportant detail; interpretations were starting to sound strange again. Some guy in a bar got aggressive with me, yelling that I was the one wandering around town with that stupid bag, yes, there it was, that stupid bag. We almost came to blows over my abrasive answer. What would normally have been an inappropriate little hostility now struck me as a typical example of the irritation I triggered wherever I went and that I hadn't noticed before. Now that I was aware of this irritation, I encountered it everywhere. A young woman approached me on the street saying wasn't I the poet at the theatre, she had a question for me. Instead of just talking to her, I nodded and fled back up the narrow street without knowing why. She called something after me, I turned around and, retracing my steps, agreed with her, not having understood a word she said. I hurried to my apartment at the theatre that was slowly turning into a daily news archive. It was full of the newspapers and almanacs I assembled and frantically rushed through, and the random issues of the *Süddeutsche Zeitung* "Diskothek" I bought, a weekly roundup of CD collections that focused on pop music highlights from 1955 to 2004. I listened to the songs again, concentrating on the years from 1977 to 1983, the period I not only found musically most interesting—postpunk, new wave, and all that—but where I also located the unspeakable betrayal I had suffered. I listened for clues in the lyrics and the melodies. This time the paranoid perspective on the world set in quickly. All I had to do was piece together the fragments of a few years earlier, and move straight back in; the paranoia was like an empty apartment, and I was once again a victim of the spirit of the world, ready to take revenge on the future. What was unspeakable was also inexpressible, and so I carried this secret around with me, like the others, not saying a word about it. These strategies were familiar to me. But it was hard to endure the inner tension.

Things soon turned pretty bizarre. "Things" here means me. Completely shaken up by the earthquake in Haiti, I crashed a rehearsal, beer bottle in hand, and sat down on the stage as though in protest. I no longer liked what they were rehearsing though I wasn't quite up-to-date. I chose to see the warning the theatre technician addressed to the director about being careful when you use water and electricity at the same time as a metaphor, since I no longer believed the laws of physics we'd learned at school. My old habit of understanding the material as metaphor and the metaphoric as material resurged. *Electricity* and *water* were words whose meanings I could no longer trust. They meant something different, but I wasn't sure what. "Yeah! Yeah!" I yelled. "Sure! electricity and water." The technician gave me a strange, almost hate-filled look, and later that evening muttered that he would have liked to punch my face at that moment. I laughed, didn't take him seriously, and by the next day had already forgotten what he and I had got so excited about.

The premiere was imminent. The team was feeling hectic, as was normal in such productions. Nerves were laid bare, also because the actors had put a lot of personal stuff into the characters over the course of the improvisations. This production in the provinces was turning into something existential, and now the author had flipped out too. At night I roamed the city, crashed a student party, talked intensely at a group of people who were willing to debate with me but soon shook me off in irritation, got into a night bus, then into a local train, fell asleep, and got woken up in the morning by the conductor who I asked where I was, was I in the Friedrichstrasse, Berlin? I could see a bleak landscape outside. Two school kids sitting behind me burst into raucous laughter and thought I was "cool." I got out, not knowing where I was. On the platform I gave the Peter Licht book I was just reading to a student. In the jargon used by emergency services when they pick up a psychologically confused person, I was already "helpless." But I was still managing to keep myself together to some extent, and even made it back to Erlangen.

7

The concept of *post-traumatic theatre* comes from the manifesto of a friend at the Prater. It refers to precisely the kind of theatre that has already replaced *post-dramatic theatre*. This theatre will work even more precisely on the trauma of the twentieth century, and in the process it will develop new advisory and programmatic concepts. Nietzsche's dictum that "if something is falling, one should also give it a push" is central to this debate. It is permitted to both dream and to rock-n-roll. And there are already plays, texts, and music that point in the direction of "post-traumatic theatre" in regard to identity and difference. The trick is that "post-traumatic" theatre works inversely and enlightens radically: it seeks to provide answers rather than entertainments. You can communicate via citations too. Antifearful texts will crisscross and hence bemoan and mock any exclusion. We can say, for example, that the supposedly anti-religious "sweat lodge" scene in the play *House to the Sun* seeks to further open up such "post-traumatic theatre" and, at the same time, to incorporate it into the canon. In general, the principle of guilt is rigorously rejected, conspiracy theories are analyzed, systems theory is poeticized. Not only a woman should always sit at the table.

Welcome, you idiots!

This text is dedicated to Sarah Kane, Aljoscha, and the Pixies.

"Manifesto on Post-Traumatic Theatre,"
January 21, 2006

8

Friends came to the premiere. A considerable drama had developed around me of which I was completely unaware. Cathy, the ex-girlfriend I'd almost got back together with over the past weeks, cried every time I turned my back on her. Aljoscha showed up as well, and burst into a short, uncertain laugh when he saw the way the books and records in my room were curated according to year of publication. Then he refused to leave my side. Other friends stood, dumbfounded and shy, around the fringes of this scene. The decision to commit me to the closed psych ward after the premiere had already been discussed and finalized. They kept it a secret from me.

I hardly registered the premiere, got slowly drunk during the performance, pulled on my stoplight-bright red pullover, which, a day later, I threw out in a rage *against everything that is put on show*, took a bow, and then headed to the room where the party would take place. I kept my whisky consumption under control and got the music started. I had been assured that I could choose the music, a task that struck me as much more existential, given the new importance of pop, than the play I was already neglecting. This play, churned out in two weeks, had set in motion a series of perceptions that totally confirmed my insights of 1999 and so fulfilled its unique function: my consciousness had reconnected with the world, which was in fact out of kilter. The play was a ladder leading to this perception and could now be kicked away. I'd almost wanted to boycott the performance. At the party I turned the music up so loud the speakers blew out.

The trip home was planned for the next day. The ambient irritation had been passed on to me and increased exponentially. Cathy and Aljoscha accompanied me through the pedestrian zone. In a sulk, I strode along in the direction of the train station, with the determination of a football player, a big bag slung over my shoulder, crashing into the occasional passerby, my face as hard as though petrified. I left most of my things in the apartment at the theatre where they were later stuffed into garbage bags I never picked up. In the train I had my first wheat beer, I smoked in the restaurant car, and scolded the waiter. An aimless aggression was throbbing through me.

When we got to Berlin, the kidnapping took place. They wanted me back in the clinic. Aljoscha was the messenger who broke the news to me over a beer in the bar in which I'd taken refuge. I didn't want to go. Anything but that. I was only now beginning to see through the world, the breakthrough was at hand, freedom was within sight. He had to let me go.

Isolation begins without the person who is becoming isolated realizing that it's happening. You're so busy, constantly out and about, meeting new people, getting involved in different groups, and creating grotesque situations. Friendly confrontation is the modus operandi of the moment, things are seething inside but it is still possible to maintain a reasonable facade. Sometimes there are meaningful silences and knowing glances, but you're not even aware of how intrusive they are.

Two other friends came by and hauled me off to the Charité, where an amiable, easygoing doctor asked me a few questions. I still didn't want to go. The doctor explained to my friends that my experiences in the psych ward had evidently been traumatic and they would have to be patient. But who can be patient with a frenetic manic? I saw how worried they looked—and gave in, agreed to stay, and a few days later discharged myself, against doctors' advice, until after further incidents I was again persuaded to enter the psych ward, which I immediately abandoned again. And so it went on, the whole year.

9

The year was full to the brim. Ding, ding, ding, ding, ding. I was suddenly nominated for prizes in three different literary genres: the Leipzig Book Fair Prize for translation, the Ingeborg Bachmann Prize for prose, and the Berlin Theatre Prize. And important publishing houses were taking an interest in my short stories, among them Suhrkamp, where I ended up, fulfilling a childhood dream. Over the first half of the year I was buoyed by this unexpected approval, which simply confirmed me in my madness. I was obviously on the right track.

In truth, I was on the worst track possible. Looking back, my public appearances were worse than mildly catastrophic. In Leipzig, where I'd been nominated for my translation of William T. Vollmann's *Whores for Gloria*, I caused a small public scandal—and in front of a large part of the literary establishment. I got into a loud altercation with the beefy security guards because I'd forgotten my invitation. I yelled and shouted and of course the louder I got the less inclined they were to let in the overwrought troublemaker in the leather jacket. "Just look at the way he's behaving," they said, until jury member Richard Kämmerlings stepped off the stage, put his hand on my shoulder, and gently led me into the room, an act for which I am still strangely grateful today. Former Austrian First Lady Frau Löffler, also a member of the jury, threw me a frightened, controlled glance, somehow obstinate. I took the seat reserved for me, feeling edgy and overexcited, but then noticed that the publishers Ulla Unseld-Berkéwicz and Michael Krüger were sitting right behind me, and although they were beaming at me in a strangely friendly way, this made me so nervous I took off, and instead, took up position at one of the high tables arranged around the edge of the hall to continue loudly mouthing off there—far too loudly—until the award ceremony finally started. As with the other nominations, I did not win. Not at all affected by this, I joined random parties in the evenings, drank everything in the minibar, and then roamed around lost in the unfamiliar city.

The theatre prize event at the Berlin Festival House saw similar behaviour. Armed with a bottle of Jägermeister, I took up a position in front of the building and in a hostile mood observed the bourgeois establishment standing around. A sinister character with a bottle in hand, in the doorway of one of the most formal cultural events, will obviously get unsympathetic looks, and I looked back even more aslant.

But I was no longer on a campaign to save the world. My megalomaniacal delusions, which saw connections everywhere, came only in occasional spurts. Still, I was sure that everyone, *every single person*, knew me, even if they didn't recognize me. This is the residue of the paranoia that a psychotic feels, leaves unquestioned, and then drags around like a ball and chain, obstructing normal movement and making half-baked lives hellish.

A director and a dramaturge from the Schaubühne, one of the places I'd always wanted to land, accepted my play for a reading; it was titled *Licht frei Haus* (Electricity on the House) and was about a dead-end group of tenants who unite in solidarity in the struggle against the government threatening to expropriate their housing. One is a student who has been suffering from mental illness, basically a stand-in for me, as so often in later works, actually as always in later works. I'd written the piece in late 2005 and personally pushed it into the mailbox of the Theatre Festival one day in the oblique beams of a friendly-cold winter sunshine, a nice moment. Now I was supposed to engage with the comments and proposed changes, but the destructive drive I felt toward my own texts came surging back and I tried, partly on purpose, partly in stupid childishness, to add as much pseudo-Dadaist nonsense as I could. The actor Jule Böwe, who was playing the main female role, asked me during one rehearsal how to pronounce a certain word that I had changed both rhythmically and semantically, and I demonstrated the pronunciation even though the word made no sense whatsoever. She nodded, thought it over, repeated it, seemed to have understood. They're used to all kinds of things in the theatre, I thought, and I still think, a notion that was supported by another rehearsal for the reading, during which the actors and the director suddenly and for no apparent reason started yelling at each other, Jule Böwe exposed her breasts, everybody else lost it, until I, the only one who was actually mad, asked them to calm down. Perhaps my own nervousness, which was already a clinical issue, had brought on their turbulence, I don't know. The tits'n'ass parts would have to go, the director told me afterward, and I just grinned and nodded. Yes, I'd given the play quite an obscene twist. Let them do with it what they wanted, I'd already moved on to other things. The reading turned out to be a solid piece of work, as you say when you don't know what else to say, and I couldn't have cared less. Somebody else won the prize, and Martin Wuttke turned to the bar in disappointment and guzzled something. I made the rounds of the groups of establishment types, drifted from here to there, drank and talked nonsense. One more festival was over, and my reputation as a crazy weirdo was further established.

It was the same in Munich that fall, at an evening of young dramatists, where I mistakenly thought I saw Elfriede Jelinek, then spent the night roaming through the streets flat broke; at some cultural breakfast in the morning I made a thundering speech into the mic attacking the absentee fathers of my generation (which greatly impressed one of the dramaturges there, as she told me after the round table—the twofold power of the manic rage is such that it sometimes hits the bull's eye), and spouted some senseless drivel onto the recorder of a culture journalist from the radio. I had no idea how drunk I was, which the journalist confirmed over the phone a few weeks later. Mission unaccomplished and in a blur, I left town, with Dirk Laucke next to me, whom I supplied with beer.

I hardly remember Klagenfurt. I'd already spent months in this state of semi-delirium brought on by psychosis and alcohol consumption, and was hardly managing to keep things together. At home, my friends held their breath as they watched the live performance on TV, worried that I might slash open my forehead during the reading, which would have been a very silly statement but representative of my frame of mind and quite unrehearsed. Or maybe I would just stand up and start shouting or ripping the clothes off my body?

I hated Klagenfurt, that much I remember; it is basically a celebration of the coterie of critics, agents, and publishers, while the authors end up standing around like cheap whores offering up their flesh to the highest bidder. I remember pushing aside one of the critics at the buffet, not in order to make more space for myself but to caricature his own pushiness. Then I strolled over to a seated group, which I knew. Charlotte Brombach, the editor, had "brought along" Josef Winkler and I was ecstatic; he was, after all, one of the literary heroes of my youth. I immediately tallied up which of his books were the best and why.

He just nodded. Many people just nodded at that point in my life. They were right to just nod. Just nod, don't say anything. I do much the same these days when I encounter crazies. I don't really know how to respond to them either.

I stormed off into the countryside on a rented bike, away from the Maria Loretto restaurant and all that crap, didn't go down to the lake for a swim, was rude to the organizer, insulted Clemens Meyer in passing, and refused to participate in anything. I hardly registered any of the competition. My new editor stayed by my side as much as she could. The song of the week, blaring from all of the speakers, was "Crazy" by Gnarls Barkley.

When it was my turn to read, I felt vertigo. The cameras were on me and I felt as though I were on a roller coaster, just at the point where it suddenly drops off. I was off-balance, everything before me was pointing downward, and then I went rattling down the slope. Still, I managed to get through the reading without incident. I just clung to the manuscript. My pace was far too fast, and in retrospect, I came across as pretty aggressively introverted, with a grotesquely gelled buzz cut—but still. I could have totally lost it.

10

I'd built one small irritant into the text, and this detail gives some idea of the twisted logic and unrealistic fantasy operating in a psychotic mind. A year earlier I had read Juli Zeh's novel *Gaming Instinct* and was amazed. I liked it, it was set in Bonn and had intelligent young protagonists who bucked authority in ways that were subversive and verging on terrifying, very good, and even better, it was written in high-speed metaphor-rich language that I was partial to. It had been a powerful reading experience that was now, in the paranoia of my manic year, undergoing change. As with most fictions, no, as with everything I encountered in the media or in person, I began to relate structures, events, and characters to myself. In *Gaming Instinct*, I now saw the main character, Alev, as a twisted portrait of myself: an intellectualized outsider from the middle of a reckless nowhere who pretends that nothing can get to him, he's beyond all morality, and decadently brilliant. There was not much that was right about this self-projection but I accepted the portrait the way I accepted everything, since in any case I was being portrayed from all sides in turned and twisted ways, and with enormous distortions, beyond my control. This Alev struck a chord in me, no, not just a chord, he set off a *drone*, to deploy a rather fat metaphor myself. Though the actual personality traits didn't quite fit, I saw my mindset reflected in an intuitively clever way, and I accepted Alev as a friend's strange but justified projection. I felt recognized. This ostensible recognition gradually blossomed into a mild and friendly obsession. In my megalomaniacal and relational madness, I figured that Juli Zeh and I belonged together, a secret set of chancellors of the underground who communicated via metaphor, which the politicians of the world were beginning to fear, but no, not just recently, ever since our childhoods when we were, unwittingly, growing up just around the corner from one another and had somehow attracted notice, tossed into this idyllic complicated Bonn that world history regarded with bated breath, this temporary capital city set up after the crimes against millions, and which was nothing more than a sleepy village on the banks of the old Rhine, whose leading role was about to be dismantled and moved to the real centres of the world.

That's what I was thinking. And I could fill many more pages with details about all this nonsense that was in my head. Sometimes I thought the sparrows on the roof were actually twittering our names and that the kids in Kreuzberg were referring to us in their role-playing, something I could hear clearly, every day, through the window.

Virtually every fixed idea that a manic has comes with a similar genealogy, a rather crazy, inexplicable origin that can, however, be narrated. Most of these ideas are frighteningly silly, and there is no point trying to unravel them.

As a way to express my gratitude for the Alev portrait, which I intensified each time I thought about it, I decided to construct a break in the fictional level of the text I would present in Klagenfurt. So instead of using the name of the protagonist Bianca in one particular spot, I uttered a heavily meaningful but somehow light, as though nudged by my elbow, "Juli." It is night, a dream scene, where the neurotic, intelligent Bianca is having a nightmare, from which my first-person narrator, also a woman, is trying to wake her up: *Bianca, Bianca, wake up.* I smuggled the foreign name into exactly this spot in the text and actually read it out loud, though against a certain inner resistance. If I remember correctly, I produced this in a particularly self-conscious and wild, uninhibited way and with an affected jerk of my head that expressed my determination to allow reality to break through fiction, and I saw this as the actual achievement of my entire Klagenfurt experience. Anyone who noticed probably found it strange. It certainly wasn't understandable. But many will not even have noticed. The video is still online. I cannot watch it. During the final copyedit of my collection of short stories which came out months later, I insisted that this wrong name be included. I wanted this window onto reality to stay open.

Some things are so embarrassing that I temporarily encrypt them in my own Word document.

11

In one of the connecting airports on the way back to Berlin, a critic wanted to take me by the hand because I'd gotten lost again. I'd managed to slip through the notoriously slippery channels of the prize-giving ceremony, but don't remember exactly how. Burkhard Spinnen had remarked that he was proud of me, but it wasn't clear to me why. Maybe because I'd made a breakthrough and established my name? Oh, and there was the editor Thorsten Arend, to whom I'd sent my entire collected works: from today's perspective, completely confused, diffuse stuff. I hope he deleted it.

A couple of weeks later I wrote Juli Zeh a polite, slightly odd email and she answered, pleasant but aloof. I was not allowed to express my actual perceptions. Those were the rules of this particular game, which didn't exist: anything that came too close to the truth had to be kept at a distance.

12

Emails. There is no form of communication that is more seductive and more pernicious for the common manic. It is just too easy to give in to sudden impulses and send a confused observation or a hastily revised burst of emotion out into the world. Something that is well-meant, or intended to cause a laugh, reaches the other side as a threat. Language is already more than a little screwy, and that intensifies the incongruencies. Language is uncertain terrain, no longer quite accessible. *Electricity* and *water* don't mean what they once meant. Idioms are systematically taken literally. Channels are shockingly open. People take potshots with images and riddles, and secrets have to be cloaked in quadrupled metaphors. Everything I send out is potentially visible to everyone else, copied thousandfold and sent

around, and what I write in an email today ends up on the
desk of the Minister of the Interior tomorrow. There you
go, I turn on the TV and see Wolfgang Schäubele, I watch
him, he actually seems to be leafing through an old version of *Saturday Night,* a sneer on his face. I have to get to
work right away to recode everything, or no, to just present everything differently, ranting and trashing it all in a
particularly determined way, no matter in what direction,
because it is my duty as a citizen and it is part of my rebel
ethos to do this here and now. The addressee whose name
is in the "send" line is not the actual addressee, and when
I write the word *Bresche* everybody knows I am indirectly
referring to "Breach," the feverish text I wrote in Austin in
1997. Even if I don't realize it myself—they always know.
All texts are fettered in tangles of references that tie my
language and my throat into knots. I have to celebrate a
desperate carnival with the letters of the alphabet and in
the process I go cryptic, but doggedly remain myself, even
if everything shifts out of line. Sometimes I have to use
words to tear the curtain to shreds. Sometimes I have to
write collective emails to bring all the lost figures together
again, under my wing, initiate projects, trigger ideas.

Emails are a disaster. A manic attack with internet access,
and you've screwed things up for life with some people. A
manic afternoon with beer, and you have once again, and
for all time, turned yourself into a freak.

13

The first set of friends gave up and turned away. I had
already lost Lukas years earlier. Things were just too difficult and hard on the nerves, too much of a shock, and they
had to take care of their own lives. My mania might fluc-
tuate but it remained a frightening and resistant constant.

And phases of fluctuation are anything but restful—for the sick person, as for those around them. The tension between acute mania and acute depression triggers aggression against yourself and against others.

Losing friends, relationships, and people who are close to you over and over again, is just unbearable, and all the more so because it far exceeds the usual rejection and alienation that life brings. This is probably why these "friends" are constantly being conjured up here, mainly as gaps, empty chairs, little illusions born of loneliness.

14

I was running out of money. Ever since Erlangen, I had been unable to carry on my freelance job as a copywriter in the oil industry, and one day I'd suddenly quit. All along it had been difficult to reconcile that work with my beliefs, and now I couldn't even make sense of the December memoranda or give them a reasonable shape. Later, at a supper with my former boss that marked my departure, she said my knuckles had been bleeding.

I started selling my books. Thomas Mann was the first to go. I'd never liked him, found his style dishonest and cloying and couldn't do anything with his famed irony. Tricks and gimmicks, sublimated pedophilia with an ancient Greek gloss—gone! The cheap collected editions of Goethe, Schiller, and Mark Twain that I'd lugged around with me since I was young—gone! Max Frisch, that senile identity stutterer and erotomaniac—gone! Uwe Johnson, the alcoholic essayist, and the two parsons, Heinrich Böll and Friedrich Dürrenmatt—gone! Almost every day I headed out to the book dealers with a heavily bulging shoulder bag and came back with little more than ten euros, which had to cover cigarettes, food, and beer. It was work, it was a workout. The emergency solution turned into a new obsession. I wanted to get rid of the books, the ballast I felt weighing me down. Literary history would continue to exist only in my mind, and besides it had turned into a history of ghosts, a spectre that was pursuing me. The books were all contaminated with messianic expectation, which—as I still believed on some days though this idea wasn't constantly present—was culminating in me. I had to clean up, clear things away, create a blank slate. Slowly my bookshelves developed gaps. I cleared out everything on analytical philosophy, deconstruction, including Foucault. My entire program in philosophy now struck me as a farce. I began to sell books that had once been important to me: David Foster Wallace, Bret Easton Ellis, Adorno, Beckett, Vollmann, Wittgenstein, Pynchon, Grass, Goetz, Zeh, Bachmann, Bernhard. Cathy begged me over the phone to at least hang on to the Nabokovs. She knew how much I loved them.

But I ended up selling them later on.

One day, one of the book dealers told me that what I was doing—the daily visits—was nonsense. If I really wanted to sell, we could just set a date for him to come by. I agreed immediately. A few days later he was in my apartment, decimating my book collection: complete works of Freud, complete works of Gottfried Benn, complete works of Joyce and Proust and Kafka, in fact, all the complete works. Peter Handke, Botho Strauss, Elfriede Jelinek—gone! Michel Houellebecq—gone! Friedrich Schlegel, Friedrich Schelling, Friedrich Schleiermacher—gone! There were no nasty intentions on his side, and I was happy, though there was some slight discomfort. But I knew that with my imminent wealth I would soon be able to reconstruct the loveliest book collection ever. Besides there were still a lot left on the shelves, even after the dealer took off with hundreds of books, the ones with the highest market value. In fact, there were still far too many left! Again, I shouldered my bag.

15

And I moved. Every manic bout brought at least one move with it. At the very least. This time I went from the Prenzlauer Berg down to Kreuzberg, right to the Kottbusser Tor. I'd ordered a Zapf moving van and three movers, which was far too much for my needs. "It's awful here," one of the movers shouted, and I didn't know if he meant Kreuzberg, or the apartment, my few boxes, or me. Aljoscha snickered frostily.

For the first weeks, I lived out of those boxes, listened to unspeakably loud music to introduce myself to the neighbourhood, and surged through the streets like a phenomenon. The summer was hot, and the midsummer pageant of the World Cup drove me ever further into madness. It was too bright everywhere, it was blinding, the flags and the banners, the TVs and the fan zones. I got aggressive, travelled back and forth through the city, sometimes yelled for Germany, sometimes for someone else, joined in football scrums on the street, kicked the ball into passing cars.

I started being a regular at a certain Kreuzberg café, or rather, I latched on like a tick. The wait staff soon got pretty tired of me, but I didn't notice or chose not to. Deep down and secretly, they were happy, I knew that, and they were safe as long as I was there. I spent the summer in this café, ignoring the occasional abuse from other customers, working on my short story collection, getting drunk, hardly eating. Slept as much as I could when I got home, and that wasn't much. Took up with a couple of women. Read the almanacs. Sold the almanacs, threw them out. There was nothing more I wanted to know, except everything.

16

Took up with a couple of women. Because it seemed so simple, and usually was too. The manic's self-confidence is enough to bring him success. He may disintegrate, but he does so with aplomb and effect. I was good at producing the greatest off-topic nonsense, which was interpreted as wit, and then rhetorical mimicry, a ban on speaking the truth, and then the gently quiet nestling up to "normal" conversation did the rest, allowing me to come across as not a totally crazy person, but rather as a crazy artist, whose strange habits were more than excusable. In classic manic-depressive manner I tended to sexual excesses and experienced myself in bed as both demonic and bestial. They'd finally bagged their Satan, their porn star, and he was performing like an overstated madman. Because he was a madman. "Is that practice, or what?" a passing fling asked. The fact that the performance was not always up to par because of the occasional medication I took I didn't blame on the medication but on the burden resting on my shoulders. After all, I had to get to the bottom of millions of discourses and histories. And under me, always the same nameless flesh.

The artist who did installations, tomboyish and quite unmoved; the woman from the gay bar Möbel Olfe who I picked up with only two sentences and who burst into laughter at the sight of my books; the lost beauty from the Roses bar, who was simply the actor Carrie-Anne Moss for me, representing a special reunion in reality because of the *Matrix* films; the acquaintance, an ex-girlfriend of a friend, which made me morally guilty; the journalist, who wanted to be mad herself; the painter; the unsuccessful lawyer; the woman without a personality from Bateau Ivre; the one without a job and with the scars below her breasts; and that one, and the other one, and her and her.

Brutality, loneliness, the attempt to use sex as a solution, almost by force. Alone, and on my way again in the morning, out from between the sheets and into the hustle of this crazy city.

17

I was a guest at Suhrkamp in Frankfurt, a publisher I'd come to see as mine and not in a healthy way; I felt downright possessive. The fulfillment of my youthful dreams had turned into a mere footnote. If the history of the world in its entire framework was coming together in me, then it was obvious that this cracked foundation of the West German intelligentsia should too. For what belonged together was now growing together, and finally united, would glow with a new brilliance. Instead of being thankful, I accepted the task of saving the publisher. Or to put it in terms of a Chuck Norris meme, I wasn't with Suhrkamp, Suhrkamp was now with me.

After a touchy-feely conversation with the editor, a disturbing visit to the theatre section, and a tour of the pragmatic sixties structure replete with history, I found myself back in the guest apartment. When I opened the fridge, someone, I think it was Frau Becker, the publisher Siegfried Unseld's secretary, said, yes, all that was for me. There were a few beers and a bottle of schnapps that I immediately christened the "Uwe Johnson Memorial Bottle," probably left behind by some previous guest. Frau Becker said goodbye, and I had arrived; I sat there undecided, tipping back schnapps. It was very West German here; really, you felt as though you were in the sixties or seventies, and the smell of the Cold War and imminent end of the world literally hung in the room, a smell of old men in the carpet, Wolfgang Koeppen giggling into his beard, Peter Handke rearing up in sudden inspiration. After I'd downed enough Uwe Johnson schnapps I headed out into the darkness of the ugly city of Frankfurt. A cook standing in front of a restaurant asked me to lend him twenty euros, which I did. He knew me, as did everyone else, and would surely pay me back. I hurried to the opera and back again. I'd rarely seen a more lifeless place. Later, in the guest apartment, I fell asleep with a cigarette in my hand, leaving large burn holes in the fine linen, which I only saw the next morning. From that point on, in my psychotic moments, including 2010, it was clear to me that Ingeborg Bachmann never died the way it was reported. It was impossible to burn to death as a result of a cigarette in bed, and even less so in the starched bedclothes of the seventies. Bachmann was alive, or she had died quietly sometime in the nineties. I called that the "Bachmann lie," and a short text I wrote about it, actually a jibe at Paul Celan, was later published in *Die Zeit*.

18

One particularly insistent tenet of my manic system was that most of the dead were still living. Death was just too sad. I saw a gallery of the undead before me and had the unshakable suspicion that many had faked their deaths because notoriety, as I had come to realize, was a killing machine. There was just too much hostility out there in the streets, in the city. Fascism suffused the air everywhere. And so somewhere, probably up in the Alps, there must be a resort, supported by Suhrkamp, to which the champions of the mind could retreat and breathe in mountain air after announcing their deaths. That's where Bachmann, Bernhard, and Beckett were. They were waiting for the moment when I would awake from hibernation. That's where Werner Schwab was, still getting drunk, and where Sarah Kane passed by on her morning run. For Bernhard, it had predictably gotten too comfortable, which was why he had apparently just fled the idyll. Or was he simply the vanguard of the next-in-line? Anyway, it's hard to believe, but I saw him once in those days sitting at the McDonald's in the Wuppertal train station, eating a Big Mac, with a grumpy expression and a skeptical sideways glance, just like on the red cover of the paperback copy of *Extinction*. He wasn't enjoying his meal. I left him to eat in peace.

The moment to awaken from my hibernation had now arrived. I was aware of my role and was sending out the appropriate signals, into the web, through letters, on the streets. As a response, I expected the arrival of the dead, their resurrection, their return from vacation. After all, Foucault was already back, one of the first, of course, and had taken over the Prater bar in Prenzlauer Berg. So the death of the author was complete, and humans were in the process of extinction like a face drawn in the sand at the edge of the sea?

But there he was, right there. And to top it off, his name was Thomas.

Right.

19

Hey! A party tonight. I've called up the right people, and they're coming over: Aljoscha, Patrick, Knut, Konrad, even Dagny. It's going to be a glamorous, unbeatable evening, we're going out to Ballhaus Ost. I dropped off some music and lyric sheets with those people before they even opened up; they're pretty bright, engaged folks. It'll be great.

We're already in the bar of the theatre. I just came from the premiere of *The Marriage of Maria Braun* and can hardly remember a thing. At most a female Hitler figure, giggling on the forestage at the start. Everything else passed me by. I'd tried to steal a beer out of the producer's fridge and got caught. That's not cool, the barman told me. I agreed. But hey! I brought you my lyric sheets along with the music on CDs I burned myself, and you made generous use of them, didn't you? Isn't that right? So is your name Pollesch? Or what? I recently had the exact same problem with him. He could have said he was just helping himself. First, you don't even confirm that the text arrived by email, and then you cite all kinds of ideas and passages. That's the way we like it! The technician rightly hissed the word *asshole* in his direction, which I heard as I left the production. It's just Pollesch, the prankster. You can't get mad at him. And besides, Hollywood's been doing this for years, so I'm not going to get all excited about a deal in this little cow town of ours called Berlin.

The music starts up and lifts me straight into abstraction. I down a beer, grab a second, distribute a whole round, and start dancing. The party hasn't really begun, but I'm feeling impatient, and wherever I am that's where the party is. That's my nature, and that's the nature of the party. My friends are standing around, kind of stiff and silent. Come on, guys! We're being liberated today! Even if it's just for a couple of hours. Let's go!

Dagny is looking really cute again. I can't remember exactly why we split up but now it feels like we're back together again. No need for words, it's enough to exchange glances, a quick touch, it's enough to be face to face. I dance around wildly, I spin her around. The lighting here has the same colours and consistency as a basement party room in the burbs, but I still feel it's just perfect, set up just right, a nice understatement. Good people. More people arrive, also good people. Only good people. I briefly talk at Anne Tismer, who laughs, intimidated. Small wonder.

At some point I kiss Dagny, it feels right, but I have to push her away again because this moment is supposed to go pop in a different way. We can kiss later. But we know. Could there be another wedding in the works, now that we've ended our hibernation? I look around. There are strangers around me, dancing, and that propels me into real euphoria. I'm dancing, they're dancing. How close strangers can get to each other. What great music this is.

The music is carrying us away, gently, into softly outlined group identities, is what I'm thinking, feeling every beat. The beat enters my head, the treble my soul, and the bass, the bass enters my legs.

Didn't pay attention for a moment, and there's Dagny in the midst of a bunch of young loudmouths, and they're leching at her. I generously ignore this. But they better not get too fresh! I'm in a heavenly mood and I don't want them getting on my nerves. But they are. I can't feel the beat anymore, and my mood collapses like the building blocks of some anemic helicopter kid in a sticker book. Hey! Hey! When I ask her, Dagny says she hasn't even noticed that these loudmouths, who are tourists, are coming on to her. Still, I hassle the tourist guys a little, toss around a few provocative gestures and words. At first, they play along, laughing. Then their faces darken. I aim a kick at them. Did I get one? I rein in my true strength.

Suddenly I'm flat out on the floor, screaming. I've never screamed like that before. One of the three just rammed his fist straight into my left eye, full force. Their first reaction was to get a little serious and plot a response, and then they answered my attempt at reconciliation with a fist to the face, out of the blue. I was smiling, and then I was on the ground. The DJ turns off the music, and only my scream hangs in the air. My friends crowd around me and make threatening gestures. Konrad says if these guys want an all-out brawl, they can have it. Aljoscha kneels to quiet me down. My eye immediately swells shut.

We take refuge in a bar, where I keep talking, my eyes closed "like a blind man," says Konrad. I must look like a broken oracle. I can't open my eye, it keeps on swelling. I keep both eyes closed because that hurts less and keep talking and talking.

Later, I sleep with Dagny, my eye shut and bloody. Why and how we got to that point, why she even went along with it, or why I did, only the devil knows.

In the streetcar the next morning, passengers stare at me surreptitiously and look shocked, my eye must look terrible, and a girl says, "Hope you get better soon," which builds me up. But I can't find my way, I wander through the snow in Prenzlauer Berg, lost in the drifts. There was a clinic around here somewhere, wasn't there? Where's the clinic? I used to know where it was, why don't I now? I sit down in the Ernst-Thälmann-Park, exhausted, and can't go on. My body is tired and cold. My eye needs to be looked at but I can't get to the clinic, wherever it is. I call Aljoscha on my cell phone, which sets off a small phone avalanche. Konrad calls Knut, Aljoscha calls Patrick, who borrows a van from Seppl. I capitulate, I cannot do it all by myself. An hour later they pick me up and load me into the van. All I want is to go to the eye clinic. But they of course have a different plan.

They take me to the Buch Clinic, where my eye gets treated. "Yes, there's this pain inside, there's this pain in the eye, and we have to get it out," murmurs the worried doctor, as she looms over me in the examining room and studies my eye close up. I don't understand why she is saying such weird things. Get the pain out? Is that a metaphor or is she just awkward?

Then we head to the psych ward in Weissensee. My friends have apparently got it all arranged, there's a spot for me. Another conspiracy. At first I resist, but then I admit defeat, and feel disappointed and hurt. They keep wanting to "deport" me, as Kevin Vennemann said. "Did they deport you again?" he asked once under the train arches at the Kottbusser Tor. Then he apologized quickly, probably scared by the expression on my face, which probably looked as though I'd burned myself.

I despise the doctor in admissions, with his wispy hair and the dumb questions on his face. He bares his teeth and seems not to understand a thing. He's just unpleasant. The reflections on his cheap glasses hardly conceal his devious eyes. Later, I discover that he advised my friends to immediately call the police if there's ever another such incident.

In comparison, my young roommate Christian is full of power and energy, talks non-stop about intelligent stuff. He is a classic manic, I can tell right away, apparently at home in every club in the city. And I believe every word. Why not? He's not making anything up.

My friends leave, they're probably exhausted. Their rescue operation, which started this morning, has taken most of the day. I eat supper and I know, nope, I'm not staying here.

The other patients ghost past me. I no longer have the resources to see them and no memory either. This time, their fates don't interest me. It's incredibly boring here.

Two days later I discharge myself and return to my wrecked apartment.

20

There's no easy answer to the question of how to protect a crazy person from himself (and how to protect others from him). The legal basis is mental health legislation, which is local. When is it appropriate to deprive a mentally ill person of their freedom, commit them, and force medication on them? The key problem here is contained in the concepts "danger to self" and "danger to others." Whoever endangers themselves or others (or the rights and property of others) and who is designated mentally ill by a doctor's certificate, can be "committed" through a local court decision, and de facto be detained. This is allegedly justified in order to maintain public order. Public order consists of all the unwritten rules that make it possible to live in society. Which brings us into the murky area of "common sense." Who spells out these unwritten laws? I have to know what kinds of legal issues can arise from my behaviour, what exactly will happen if I disturb the public order—that is what our so-called principle of legal certainty prescribes. And there is much that is "unwritten." Basically, those are limits that are based on feeling, not facts.

Surely, I can buy whatever I want. Some people incur debts merely for tax reasons. And isn't the economic system equally manic and irrational when it feverishly piles up debt and views the future as a wager? You just don't know what it's betting on.

Did the time I spent in psych wards ever prevent me from doing anything? Or anything worse? Maybe it did; I can't know that. The damage afterward was so enormous that what were once traumatic stays in psych wards soon felt like harmless little excursions. No, they didn't achieve a thing. Or maybe yes: they let everyone else briefly take a breather. But it was other factors that helped me regain my health.

Besides, what exactly does this mean: crazy, mentally ill? I think murder is so crazy I would formally certify the madness of any murderer. And thereby oddly absolve them of their guilt.

When a Germanwings pilot deliberately crashed a plane in the French Alps in 2015, thereby killing 149 people, I followed the public discussions closely, combing through the reports and accounts every day, analyzing the premature judgments and arguments. And how dishonest I was to hope the perpetrator, whom I definitely believed to be bipolar, would just be labelled depressed rather than subject to what I still think was wrong with him.

I have been a danger to myself, though not to others. Others have found me totally irritating, and some have found me frightening. I can agree with all that. I simply want to point out how murky the legal situation is. There are unpredictable moments. And none of the efforts expended heal the mania; they just muffle it, sideline it. The border between help and control is fluid, which makes it all so complicated and sensitive.

Another issue is the undignified manner in which you are turned into an object of the bureaucracy. The privatization and capitalization of the health and social services sectors make the marginal person a product that can be milked. Suddenly, people you wouldn't normally acknowledge, even in a half-assed way, are pushing you around, small-minded, worn-out functionaries who impose the minuscule, decaying vestiges of their power on you, all the while keeping profits in mind. They can't afford to lose money, they're beholden to the bottom line.

And if you don't comply, they clamp down slowly and mercilessly, like those old metal brackets in ring binders. The bureaucratization of the systems that were originally designed to help adds so much randomness and so much inhumanity to the situation that anyone who has escaped these forces must wonder how they ever got away.

But what other solutions are there?

21

The wounds healed more slowly, the scars accrued more quickly. There were more stays in clinics, more attempts to confine me, Haldol treatments, self-motivated discharges. The time drew near ... But which time? I didn't know that I was sick; ironically, I revised a couple of pieces about my 1999 bout for *Raumforderung*, my first collection of short stories, fixed a word here and a word there, thrilled by the precision I was able to attain. I churned out another two or three pieces that at times made no sense at all, and only related the crassest details, like "Kippy Game 2." Indeed, I was then obsessed with Martin Kippenberger, also one of the undead, who I thought I'd spotted in the Morena Bar. I bought a photo book, an exhibition catalogue, and two scholarly works about him, read them in a scattered kind of way, wrote and scribbled in them, laughed myself silly, and saw my own hysterical-alcoholic activities mirrored in his works and life. Where was he now? There he was! Over there! Gone again. Oh, they were all coming to help me out, they were still there, those good, old, undead spectres.

I started drawing again, obsessively. As a young student I'd done some painting and drawing, mostly faces, sometimes urban scenes, focusing on technique first, and then on distortion. Now I wanted to extravagantly live out my talents as an all-round artist, painting wherever I could, using a copy of the *taz* to compose a remix of Kate Bush's newest album *Aerial* (nice that she was back again from her fortress; I was so happy, many greetings!), I left the *taz* lying at the San Remo Upflamör, and that evening recognized the remix in a DJ set by T. Raumschmiere. The way everything was connected! Thank god they hadn't kicked me out of Maria, the way they recently had out of Blumfeld and Mia. At Blumfeld a security guard just grabbed me from behind, lifted me up, and carried me off; I hollered, I let loose a loud yell, and Distelmeyer interrupted the concert he was giving. At Mia, in Hamburg again, the doorman threatened to break both my arms. That's no way to do your job, guys. In my room in Kreuzberg, referred to as my "studio"—much like the psychotic in Sven Regener's *Herr Lehmann*—I created a sculpture out of some clothing, an iron, paints, duvet feathers, clothes hangers, and newspapers that at some point turned out to resemble a mouselike monster. A mouse? What was *that* supposed to mean? Snip, I shortened the electrical cable on the iron, tail gone, mouse dead. A Turkish neighbour across the way watched all this skeptically, and then closed her window, which was covered with aluminium foil, forever, it seemed to me.

A fit of rage soon took hold of me, for no particular reason, and I tore the sculpture to pieces. Then I carved a double version of Beethoven's destiny motif from the Fifth Symphony into the wallpaper above my bed. It had no effect. Then I started to hurl books and records out the window. Because I was angry with them, these products of the mind and the creative spirit. Boundless vampirism! The things crashed and bashed into the courtyard below, and made a lot of noise; for about five minutes I threw whatever I could get my hands on onto the asphalt and into the bushes in a great rage, until I finally realized that this did no good either. Not even a single neighbour came to complain. I closed the window. Hours, maybe a day later, I picked up the things I'd thrown out, stuffed a few of the books I still liked into my backpack, and tossed everything else in the garbage.

And continued my trembling rounds as a fool.

22

A trip to Hamburg, with Hans Magnus Enzensberger disguised as a woman in the next compartment. Was that supposed to be clever? So Enzensberger-clever, always a step ahead? What a smartass! He's annoying. That morning I'd already seen Alexander Kluge in front of the chancellor's office, turning, smiling. Putting out a calmer vibe than he did in his DCTP TV broadcasts.

But now it's Hamburg, I'm drawn there every time I've understood the truth. Storming along the Outer Alster Lake. Realizing my leather jacket is bait for swans. The swans follow me as I head toward the centre. The beauty and grace of these birds, no wonder Hölderlin succumbed to madness at the sight. Suddenly I hate the leather jacket and stuff it into a garbage can. Hope the swans die. But it's cold without my jacket, where is it warm? I tear around like a madman, and somewhere I find a bar with scraggy grey heroin figures. Are those really whores? Get talking to a transvestite who looks strangely like one of the patients from the Urban Hospital. Why are we being brought together? He gives me a blow job. Or do I just imagine that? I watch sado-masochistic games, a man in the street on a chain like a dog, he's being hauled along on a studded choker, his skin pallid and splotchy. Disgust, confusion, outta here. It's better on the Sternschanze, through the bars and pubs there. Had some strange conversations. Got on somebody's nerves? Absinthe. Can't keep going. Rented a room in a flophouse on St. Georg, hardly slept. I can't sleep when I'm dead either. Short breather: scraps from the past. Here, in this area, I was happy exactly twice. But there's none of that now.

Got on the wrong train and fell asleep, arrived in Oldenburg. What am I doing in Oldenburg? A fit of rage, and my fist slams into the digital noticeboard between the train cars, which unfortunately shatters. I stand in front of the Oldenburg train station like a statue. Carstensen, the politician, who is looking for a wife with the help of the *Bild* newspaper, hurries past (or is it a doppelgänger?), and hisses an obscenity at me. Just as I understand what he's saying, a couple of policemen rush me. I don't budge an inch. They put me in a police hold and drag me over to the wall, push me hard up against it, although I am not resisting, and tell them so. They struggle to get handcuffs on me. I tell them I'm coming along. They can't get the damn handcuffs around my wrists, scrape open my skin in the process. They must be more flustered than I am. Finally, they're on. I'm led away through the train station, spotlight on me, surprised glances, to the police station. They take down my personal details.

"Why do something like that, Herr Melle?"

I shrug.

"This will take its usual course."

They let me go, I don't care, I could just as well land in the notorious drunk tank even though I'm not drunk. Instead, I'm back in front of the train station, as motionless as before. Damnoldenburg! Where to? Totally lost. Ask a taxi driver about hotels. We check out three or four, there's nothing available, apparently. He doesn't know what's up either, offers to drive me to Bremen for a special price. This happened to his son once too. I accept, grateful.

Bremen, some hotel room. I try not to leave a trace, don't know why. Suddenly I'm a spy, all churned up, push-ups and television. Watch the street through the slit in the curtains. Eat a light but pretentious breakfast. Am stupid, but clever.

From an internet café (with Gary Oldman beside me, completely drunk), I send out a proposal for a collaborative play to eight female and male playwrights, to be written collaboratively by everybody and including everything. Over the course of the day some of the recipients actually answer and even discuss possible themes. I am ecstatic, really pleased with the team spirit, and I expect the best play since '45.

Catch up with myself in Wuppertal, celebrating the "triumph of the provinces." Sit on a slope with a can of pop, staring at the cable cars, and phone my editor, as though she were Miss Moneypenny—charming and mysterious. Later, the same nutty idea: I leave the hotel room exactly the way I found it. Not a trace, not a *single* trace. That's fun. I take the key with me. It's all mine anyway, or will be soon, or sometime.

Stop in Bonn briefly, my mother is afraid of me. I smash the glass of a framed portrait of Günter Grass that I sketched at the age of fourteen and he wrote a comment on, tear up the portrait, and toss the scraps off the balcony into the garden. He should be ashamed of himself, that ss henchman.

In Berlin I almost die when I see an acquaintance on the other U-Bahn platform, stupidly take a step toward him, and fall down onto the rails. The U-Bahn is still far away. I almost die another time when I ignore the traffic on the Warschauer Bridge and almost walk into a speeding car. "One more step, and you'd have been gone." Two young guys laugh in shock. That evening I crash a gallery, ask a senseless question about Kippenberger in the discussion that is taking place about computer games and art, and disrupt the concert that follows. A woman curator hisses at me—one more word and she'll "fuck" me. The band ends the concert when I smash a glass.

Days later, back in Hamburg, I make my way up a steep hill beside a fairground, dig my fingers into the dirt, shovel my way up. I have to get rid of the boundless power in me. At the top, I look out over the city. Am I growing wings? I leap in my thoughts, I leap for real. Nothing. What am I looking for? I tear down the slope, slip and slide. Later, in Berlin, I label the dirt on my runners "yon soil from Hamburg," laughing, and people join in laughing.

23

Hamburg is an obsession and a symptom: if I don't have an appointment but am in Hamburg anyway, you can assume it's a manic phase. Hamburg attracts me when I'm stuck, spinning around in psychotic loops. I accuse the city of being my actual home. Where does this yearning for Hamburg come from? The openness, the citizenry, the Hamburg School, the port? The years get mixed up too. Sometimes I don't know what belongs to 2006 and what to 2010. I had to think about it with the swans, but now I know: it's obvious, it was 2006. Or was it? Yes. Right? Right.

Maybe Hamburg, because my supposed internet love from 1999 came from there. In my manic bouts there's always the urge to go back to the places where it all started: Bonn, Hamburg, the web, the forums. Like an arsonist who has to go back to where he committed his crime—except that for me there's a delay of several years. Or it's an unconscious craving for the time before the attacks.

Main station Hamburg, again and again, the notices flicker, I buy an Aphex Twin CD at Karstadt, visit the Thalia bookstore, wander around, Richard Powers ambles by, hello. I just brought a family I vaguely know homemade whisky chips in Johnny Cash CD covers. Back to the train station, missed another train. It's not so easy to travel in this confused condition, and catch the right train to get you home, it's not easy to constantly mix up the platforms and not lose it in a fit of rage and impatience. Getting there works well, getting back is hell. In the end you've missed all the trains and spend the night shivering on some park bench. In 2010 I spent three entire days like that in Vienna.

Then, finally, back in Berlin. Constantly on the go there, not a lot of money, quite a few restraining orders, but still not enough. The thing with the Blumfeld concert sticks in my mind. How come it was precisely this band that saw me kicked out, and not even Distelmeyer stepped in? Even Kool Savas stayed cool when I yelled for him to get back onstage! I find out the name and address of the Blumfeld concert organizer in order to sort that out. He's right around the corner. I go and get into a pretty loud yelling match with a beefy guy, one of the employees gets fed up and mediates. Days later when I show up at the Strokes for the concert, she's at the cash and says, "Oh, you again." She takes a short pause and then says, "I'm inviting you to the Strokes." No incident there, just beauty and guitars.

I despair, but still haven't had enough. Christmas is coming, the year's almost over, the book is done, my strength is waning. At the publisher's they're organizing an event with three other authors, *Nothing friendly about us*, or something like that. It's okay, it's okay.

I go to Bonn. I hate Bonn so much, and still I have to go. The book about where I came from—I'll only be able to write it in ten years or so, if ever. I arrive, everything is so small again, so yesterday. I have the great idea of taking a hotel room in Godesberg—still a sort of spy idea, to be there *undercover*, with nobody knowing officially. It'll get around anyway. In Bonn, I'm obsessed with Juli Zeh again, think I see her everywhere. We're in charge here, *Aggro Bonn*, or something like that. I laugh, and check into a rather unsplendid hotel on Koblenzer Strasse.

At six in the morning I'm sitting straight up in bed, sleep is out of the question. I check out, have a coffee at the baker's and eat a croissant. Interesting how thin I've got, there in the reflection in the window. This city drives me nuts. Traffic-calmed and recently Middle Easternized. I have a new idea, and decide to visit my old school, up on the hill. The socialization I experienced there, the way the proletarian kid was educated out of his not-self-imposed immaturity, the opportunities that opened up for me there, à la Johann Gottlieb Fichte—a visit would be a good thing, logical and appropriate. I don't want to see or meet anyone, I just want to be there on the grounds and feel those vibes. The time is right.

24

School was what saved me. But that's also where the failed *Bildungsroman* that runs through this entire book sets in. At first though, in the first two years of school, that were tyrannized by what I suspect was an old Nazi principal, I learned to love learning. An alternate world opened up for me where I could get away from the narrowness and the brutality of home, at least for a time, and free my head. I began to love school, the letters of the alphabet came flying toward me. Excited and happy, I copied them onto paper that had more lines on it every year, and early on I decided to be a doctor someday, to cure something. But the letters were stronger, and later, in high school, they came bundled up in stories written in Latin, the old-new language that let me feel part of a tradition and that was completely foreign to my background. I wrote my first poem, "Ode to Coal," about the coal I'd lugged up from the cellar for years, and I realized that the ambiguity of this song of praise about an experience I'd found humiliating made the past shimmer and almost exorcized it. So that was now mine, something no one could take away, and the infection of language and fiction gripped me even more. At the same time, I was getting official recognition at school, growing a kind of identity: a child of the proletariat was the best student among upper-class and aristocratic kids—but I was constantly on my toes. Any acts of teenage coolness or rebellion had to have a certain content and academic brilliance. For a start, I became invulnerable on all sides and let nobody get at me anymore. Only words.

Beyond the social aspects there was always some sort of escapism involved: an addiction to TV as a child; then to comics, heaps of them; then astronomy, I spent a whole winter outside between the housing blocks with a map of the stars in hand. Then all the detective fiction, along the lines of *The Three Investigators*, everything from Karl May to Jules Verne and on through the much-admired book collection of a distant uncle, landing early on *Homo Faber*, Brecht, and *The Tin Drum*. I was done for. It was decided. That was *exactly* what I wanted and what I would do, the way was clearly marked.

Normally, a boy of my background would be advised to head in other professional directions if he had the chance. Middle-class professions in law or medicine were solid and meant a leap upward, didn't they? Or how about television?

But that was not what I wanted, or what I was even capable of. I wanted to be a writer. The fact that there are also crass class differences in the realm of literature was something I didn't yet grasp, and if I had an inkling my acquired arrogance let me ignore it.

At the time my mother was working half days as a secretary in a small publishing house that produced pop psychology, so I got a discount on books. I bought and read everything. And I always asked for and usually got collected works for the various birthday and other celebrations. I never stopped reading. There was no comparing what I read to the life around me. It was simply the most amazing thing that had ever happened to me. But life still played the biggest role in these books, deals were made, broken, reflected, and the ugliest turned beautiful. That's exactly it, I thought, that and nothing but that.

And then suddenly there was theatre. I attended the plays put on by the Bonn Schauspiel, where a young Wolfram Koch appeared onstage; I didn't understand too much of it and felt intimidated by the upper-class bearing of the other people present, but I felt I was in the right place, close to an excitement machine I could connect to and get charged up by. A further world to investigate. I began to direct plays at the Jesuit academy that vigorously promoted me, and toward which I was now headed as I made my way up the hill in a manic condition. And since my mother had no resources with which to deal with my puberty, except hysteria, the principal helped me get a scholarship that allowed me to spend the last two school years there as a boarder. The fact that it was precisely this academy that was later embroiled in a child-abuse scandal is a story that has already been told elsewhere (and needs to be told some more). If I was touched by this it was only in a very fleeting way as my love-hate relationship with that place, which later crumbled underfoot, brought on a re-evaluation of my entire youth. For the time being, however, I was simply grateful, without giving up my pride, I made full use of the opportunities and perfected a crude combination of conformism and rebellion—which continues to this day.

This was where it all began and I wanted to make a brief return visit.

25

I am stomping up the hill through the Redoutenpark and thinking about the Jesuits' loyalty to the pope. The secretive, centuries-long behaviour of the Jesuits, their conspiratorial aspect, also has something to do with me. But today I don't care. Today is my day off. A couple of boys are at the entrance gate, and so are two men. It's almost eight o'clock, the last day of classes before the holidays, it seems. I walk up the first section of the Petersbergstrasse, and let that name "Petersbergstrasse" resonate in my head, and also "Elisabethstrasse," and I remember how, in the head of the child I used to be, these words changed from abstract, fearful concepts to establish themselves as common street names. I'm almost through the gate. A third man appears out of nowhere and indicates that I should stop, which I do. A gentleman wearing glasses steps out of the gatehouse, probably a teacher, and peers over at me. The men glance at him, he points at me and nods. Then he disappears. The men grab hold of me and ram me hard up against the gate. *Hey, what's all this?*

"Hands up!"

Is this a movie?

I don't struggle, I'm getting used to this kind of thing. I'm carrying two shoulder bags, I'm loaded down, which

I now realize may make a strange impression. There are books, CDs, a computer, toiletries in those shoulder bags. There are books and CDs in the pockets of my jacket as well. They empty my pockets, and the cop doing so doesn't take care, he demonstratively drops everything on the ground, the books get scratched up and smeared, the CD cases break open.

"What's going on?"

"Quiet."

"Be careful with my stuff!"

No reaction. A fourth cop in uniform is sitting in a car, with the door open, his police pants are stretched tight over his fat thighs. He gapes at me stupidly and waits. Herr Aufenanger comes out of the school, I recognize him, the music and philosophy teacher, a sophisticated mind.

"How are you, Thomas?"

He doesn't seem to believe what's happening.

"All good, Herr Aufenanger, as you can see."

I'm still up against the gatehouse wall, my hands pressed on the stone, and the cop is fumbling around in my back pocket. Another policeman steps up to Aufenanger and whispers something.

"So, now you want to make *me* a suspect? You want to arrest *me*? You've got some nerve!" Aufenanger exclaims angrily. He nods at me again, but gets pushed back and is forced to leave.

Somewhere behind me, at a safe distance, a couple of school kids are enjoying the show, among them my cousin Hendrik, as I later learn. We don't recognize each other.

It takes an hour for them to finish. Handcuffs on, and off. I don't understand why. Finally, a vestige of normal human emotion, as well as the recognition of legal rights prevails and I ask what I am accused of.

"We'll clear that up at the station."

Then I drift off again. I tell myself there is probably some reason for what's happened, after all I am the most perfidious messiah of all time, and I do indeed have ideas that are hostile to the state. They're welcome to briefly arrest my spirit. I am clever enough to ensure they can't really find anything on me. They're welcome to take a close look, this is a minor exercise for me after all the terror I've already lived through this year, and no salvation in sight.

26

They take me home to the Haribo slums. I'm supposed to have done something on the internet. Again? Apparently I published a threat against my old school. Which I didn't. My mother is completely distraught and assures them that I would never do such a thing. That's not me! She's in tears. How often do police investigators show up in your doorway, look around, interrogate, question you! They refuse to be appeased and take me to the police station. I resort to inner immigration. I've got Joachim Fest's *Not I: Memoirs of a German Childhood* with me, just in case.

What if they twist the facts? I remember Vollmann and his knowing grin when he told me that the "internet is evil. They change the data." And it's true, they could make all kinds of allegations, manipulate and change everything, and turn it against me. I am at their mercy. And didn't they just recently, on May 1, in fact, beat me up to the point of concussion? They're capable of anything.

The wait at the station is endless. The policeman with the face of a lizard and the deeply etched dark green circles under his eyes ostentatiously takes off his revolver, gives me a long meaningful look, and in slow motion locks it away in a safe under the writing desk. He's in full threat mode. Meanwhile, I am reading *Not I,* just as ostentatiously, and have put on my most arrogant face.

"Herr Melle, you make me mad," he says, and he means it, dead serious.

27

It really wasn't me. No matter how crazy I was, I knew what I'd done and what I hadn't. Weeks later it turned out that some teenager in the Bergisches Land region had uttered the threat in a chat room. The boy didn't even have anything to do with the school. But chance had led me into the arms of the police—after a stupid night in a hotel, tramping along laden with shoulder bags, psychotic and crazy—just when the cops were expecting a potential shooter. And for a few hours everybody thought the moment had come. I'd become an assassin.

The avalanche of phone calls began. The threat had made the radio news, as had the announcement, hours later, that a suspect had been arrested. While my friends were phoning the school, conferring among themselves, not believing it, but also believing it, I was already in jail. The police checked through the files in my computer, dug through my wallet, searched everything. The police station was like a comedy show: "Hey, Frau Fenstermeister, not like that, not like that!" "That's how we like it, partner!" and other kinds of ragging. They slurped the typical cop coffee and made typical cop jokes. "We're in the *Power Centre* here," I was advised in a whisper that was both threatening and ironic. The lizard was not on my side, but his colleague with the curly, thinning hair was. His son went to the same school. They accused me of having some problem with the school. I must have implied something like that earlier when I chatted casually about my past, unaware of how serious the situation really was.

The waiting, the glances, restless legs. Policemen come in, ask questions, leave. "Not me." Hours go by.

"Wasn't him! Just wasn't him!" the cop with the curly hair suddenly yells in a local accent down the thickly-carpeted corridor. Which is what I'd told them right from the start.

They kept my computer over Christmas and dropped me off at the psychiatric ward of the Rhineland Clinic.

"Oh, so you're friends now?" the lizard muttered to Curly on the way there, when we exchanged a few non-hostile words. I didn't say anything more after that.

The gateman looked up from his paper.

"Yes, hello. Police, criminal investigation. We're dropping someone off."

28

Doped up again. Haldol, parked in the smoking room. A small Trent Reznor look-alike noticed how angry I was, flung up his arms, and pushed the alarm button on the colourful wall. It was only painted on. He stood there in front of it for five minutes and couldn't figure it out. Kept pushing the painted button.

My aunt brought me a bar of soap and some cigarettes. She sniffed at the soap. She knew the place.

29

Years later I made a list of all the violations the police committed against me and published it in the summer 2010 issue of *Dummy* magazine, which appropriately had "police" as its theme. I've always known what belongs where. I still have a copy. On the second and third pages, I lay out eight or nine points in edgy handwriting while the middle of this double page spread is dominated by an advertisement for a clothing store called Herr of Eden; I also note the amount of money I claimed in a manic demand for compensation, a total of around one million euros.

I still think that, all in all, this is justified.

30

You can imagine the weeks of collapse that followed and were accompanied by a descending soundtrack, dissonant strings, the ringing of synthesizers, that all described a dogged downward movement. Mania lapped over into the new year but grew more porous. I met with people I knew in Berlin and told them about my experiences, laughing indignantly. It made me angry. I was innocent. Nobody understood me, only Gunther said, "All you wanted to do was pay your old school a visit!" Exactly, exactly that kind of sentence, and your so-called soul briefly breathes free.

I met Yvonne: two totally twisted psyches, temporarily entangled. Beers quickly chugged allowed me to brighten up once again but I soon saw that the energy they provided was on loan. The darkness of the city became almost physical and hampered my steps. The apartment? Strange, what had I been looking for here, why had I moved here? And the feathers all over the place, and all the patterns scratched onto the walls.

The paranoia dissipated, the last bits of my delusional network of relations fell apart. My usual coherence returned, but with it a silence, a paralysis that numbed body and soul. It got even quieter, and my thoughts and feelings were blunted. The noise of the bathroom ventilation pushed its way back into my consciousness; another apartment, the same effect. It roared into action whenever I stepped into the bathroom, carrying an eerie hint of extermination. I remembered the sound. It reminded me of the downward spiral that would end in nothing. After days of concealing my condition to the outside and a simultaneous quiet withdrawal into a muffled inside, it took only hours for me to realize what had been so obvious to everybody else for the past year, what they could so clearly see and what was now suddenly clear to me too: the catastrophe. The whole year had been a catastrophe. I was a catastrophe.

Things went black.

31

Nutella and cigarettes, Yvonne wrote in her journal, *he lies there and lives on Nutella and cigarettes*. I thought it was indiscreet and tactless to write such stuff. But I was helpless, and to write is to betray, also to betray yourself. Who knows that better than the writer of these lines?

Down, down: *down*. There was nothing left to keep me here. The apartment at the Kottbusser Tor was a stranger's, and there were feathers everywhere, I couldn't get rid of them, I must have slit open a whole duvet. The books were gone, the neighbourhood scorched. I avoided my friends. I would slink to Kaiser's, maybe buy some groceries—milk, pop, Choco Pops—and slink back. Try to clean up a little.

Once again the neuronal processes of depression were made worse by heavy feelings of shame, frightening memories of the recent past. I wanted to sink into the ground. I wanted to disappear. Every hour suicidal ideas would intrude, hang there, coat all other thoughts, lurk in the background, and finally settle as the dark reason for every movement.

Aljoscha sat there facing me at my writing desk and reading the *Die Tageszeitung*. I couldn't understand why it was making him smile, what kind of pleasure such a paper could bring. I could no longer grasp or understand anything.

The publication date of *Raumforderung* was approaching. It triggered nothing in me, no feeling, no joy, even though everything was coming together, everything I'd ever wanted. When the package with my copies of the book arrived, I almost wanted to cry. So it did trigger something: a meta-sadness at the realization that I couldn't feel happy anymore about anything, and that even the ways in which writing made life appealing had been lost. I leafed through the book and didn't know what to do next. It was the loss of everything here and now, and it would never be any different.

Almost as an alibi, I started on the translation of Vollmann's *Europe Central*, which I'd agreed to do. But I only got to page 3. I literally broke down before the monster text. Where'd my internet gone? Turned off.

Then the Leipzig Book Fair, where the book was launched. I couldn't go, called in sick. I devoured antidepressants, which had no effect. They never work for me. Or yes: the side effects. The days stalled. The days began with a negation and ended with a capitulation.

I did make it to one event: a book launch held in the Red Salon at the Volksbühne Theatre with three other young Suhrkamp authors. I felt obliged and gathered all my strength, downed a bunch of anti-anxiety pills in order to, perhaps, maybe utter a few weak words. Oddly enough, and it was much the same at the book launch for *Sickster* in 2011, I made it through passably well despite depressions and an extremely dark disposition, and was able to produce answers to questions from some pop literature researcher in semi-witty stanzas that struck me as a mendacious, prefabricated extension of the book, broken into textual modules. The low point that I was speaking from together with the medication let me sound more casual, breezier than I would have in supposedly healthier times. A sad form of freedom.

Nothing happened. It went on: another day, and another one, and another one. I dragged my way through time, ever more burdened, lumpier, resistant.

It didn't turn out the way you wanted it to
It didn't turn out the way you wanted it to, did it?

32

My head has the not-so-strange peculiarity of suddenly playing some random song. I may see an image, read a line, hear a motif or a name, and be set off. Then I head through the streets with the so-called earworm, unaware of it, and it accompanies me as a constant remix, looping as I write, read, eat. Gradually, I become aware of the playback, and usually wonder where this particular song came from.

"Fernando" by ABBA has a special place in this playlist. It's strange, because I don't like the song, it's too sweet, too slow, too ABBA. But in one particular situation it floated to the surface, out of the distance, like a forgotten childhood melody.

I cringe a little at describing what follows; there are no disgusting details but the whole thing is somehow shameful in its intimacy.

Of course it has to do with a suicide attempt, a half-hearted one that didn't succeed. *Succeed, crowned by success, achieved the desired result*—words with such positive connotations are not appropriate here. Nothing "succeeds" here. *Success* is not a word suited to such descriptions, and it is very debatable whether a final exit truly fulfills the "wish" of a suicidal person, even if you support a person's right to choose an uncomplicated and painless death, as I do. Further, the subtext of such language implies that the person who has not been "successful" is weak and incapable: they can't even get their exit right.

I was afraid. I didn't want to throw myself in front of a train. I didn't want to jump down from somewhere either and end up in a bloody mash. These options struck me as too martial and drastic, and also too inconsiderate. Besides, I wouldn't have the courage to take the final step. These reservations, which anyone plagued by such thoughts probably has, images of wheelchairs, leg stumps, and quadriplegic paralysis—no thanks. But I really wanted to be gone. That yearning was strong, even if I kept on, doggedly, enduring the pain and not getting rid of it. And maybe it would all come back one day—life, and the feeling of life?

For the totally desperate person, forums on suicide—please excuse my point of view, which is not meant to be cynical, quite the contrary—are a distraction. It's almost like watching TV; you zap around in them and forget yourself. In fact, after visiting such a site, you're in much the same boat as those others assembled there who are all in search of an exit strategy—you're ten times more lost than you were before, which is not the worst thing for survival. In a perverse kind of way, you even feel entertained and understood. There are detailed descriptions of bizarre ways to commit suicide: suffocation as a result of barbecuing in a bathroom that has been completely sealed off is hard to believe; gas masks, overdoses of water, all that and more, I will spare you the details. A few hours have gone by, and for the moment the question *Yes, but how exactly?* has dissipated the pain.

I found out that the active ingredient in an over-the-counter painkiller, if taken in large quantities and retained for a day, would lead to irreparable liver damage and then, within three or four days, to a painful but definite death. This information had been circulating on the web for some time, and so the company had reduced the size of the packages in which it sold the pills to packs of ten tablets. Nowhere did it say that death through the intake of these pills was actually pretty unlikely. Or I was just too dim to read and understand.

I started making the rounds of the pharmacies to collect a big supply of these pills. I was in no great hurry. I wasn't sure either if I would actually take them. But I wanted to have them, and hoard them, and I stashed them under the kitchen sink. As soon as I had the strength I would act.

And then, and here we're getting to ABBA's "Fernando," there was a cable hanging down from the top of the thermostat of my bathroom heater. I had knotted a loop into it. There was no other place in the apartment where I could somehow attach a rope, and I didn't have the strength to go out into the woods and find a suitable branch. And so I tested out my death in the bathroom. I wanted to get closer and closer to the edge. And maybe beyond it.

I am no longer able to reach back into that condition of gloomy proximity to death even though I was the one who was vegetating and dying. I can't really make it plausible to myself, so how can I do so for you?

But yes, now I remember. I remember a glance at a ledge in the Potsdamer Strasse. I remember the meaningless light. I remember how brittle time and space felt, the weight of emptiness, the rustle of my jacket as I walked. I remember every single dragged-out step. The heaviness of my lungs, the numbness of my appendages, the lack of belief in my own fate. The feeling I already knew of not belonging to the same species as others, sent off by them to live in a splintery gap, just not living anymore. I remember the total outside-it-all.

And in writing this down, I feel that way again.

The suicide techniques I described above are referred to as "soft," and statistically are preferred by women. In terms of suicide techniques I am a woman, and the attempts I have survived can be described as "appellative." They are cries for help, so I'm told. But it's not so simple, because the will to be gone is there and stronger than everything else. It's just that you don't want to end up as a hunk of useless flesh or disabled if your attempt fails.

An acquaintance used the word *coward* to label the Swiss André Rieder, who was manic-depressive and ended his life with the support of the euthanasia group Exit. The documentation about him is available on YouTube. But why is he a "coward"? Why this traditional notion of manhood, of resolve and the consequences of an action? Women are allowed to take poison, and men are supposed to throw themselves onto a circular saw? Then I opt to be a woman. It's probably really courageous to take that last step and leap off a high-rise building. But I'm unwilling to condemn someone for not doing that. I do not see why someone who has spent twenty years in painful martyrdom, brooding over a decision, and who resorts to poison in order to exit life should be considered a coward. Surely their decision is more thought through and more humane than a sudden death blow.

(By the way, the picture of André Rieder is far more typical of a bipolar person than the haggard, nervous, and always feverish clichéd image: he was described as a round "bear of a man," a slow and also physically worn colossus, with something of a civil servant or insurance salesman about him, and who hardly showed any emotion in his swollen face; meanwhile strong emotions were what had destroyed his life. Kay Redfield Jamison wears a similar expression, her feelings barely discernible. And Sinéad O'Connor, who made public her bipolar diagnosis in 2007 and retracted it in 2013, and who was once one of the most beautiful women around, now looks completely frumpy. It is no accident that people's faces grow coarse, look armour-plated and emotionless; it tells of the many deaths these people have died, and not only internally.)

I tried to avoid rope marks on my neck. Things often turned black as I huddled there with my weight hanging in the loop, dragging me into semi-consciousness, as I thought about the terrorist Red Army Faction women in Stammheim who'd also brought about their end this way (or had they?). And then the ventilation, the cynical, automatic ventilation, always there, and the white tiles round about me.

Once I was already far over the edge. My blood was stalled, my brain was stalling. And that song "Fernando" came to me. I now know where from: years earlier, Cathy had admitted, laughing, how much she liked it, and we'd listened to it together, both delighted and alienated. I'd never thought about that song again, and now that I was hardly there anymore, I heard it, it resonated like a last greeting from life into the realm of the dead. I heaved myself back up out of the blackness that had already dragged me down and swallowed me, and breathed in. The light returned, my blood circulated, my brain rebooted. Confused, I lay there on the bare floor, and couldn't understand what the song was telling me. Meanwhile it was pretty obvious: images of a harmoniously shared life, a time when life was open and on the right track. At the last moment, the possibility of a happy life had shoved its way into my dying consciousness through a song I didn't like, a flat fluffy pop promise that suddenly felt as right as nothing else had. I breathed deeply and got up, letting the song play on in my head. Then I dismantled the cable contraption and threw it away. Not like that.

This time there were rope marks. My narcissistic therapist didn't see them, and I never went back to him.

33

I'd never gone in much for therapy, which my circle of friends considered reckless. Someone like me, and no therapy? Irresponsible. I'd always resisted psychoanalysts and other psychobabble or silent treatments. It was enough to see who subjected themselves to such a massaging of the soul: almost everybody. At least in Kreuzberg, where I'd lived for a long time. People would pimp their biographies up to the heights of ancient myths, clip Electra complexes to each others' lapels, and feel like Oedipus. Everyday conversations turned into highly complex mirrorings, and a pub crawl quickly became a meditation. Instead of facing their conflicts they scurried off to the therapist in whose office their own version of the thing could be inflated and confirmed. And so they turned into ego-ish little critters. They twisted endearing personal quirks into highly meaningful human epics, and inflated them into the plot points of a psychodrama that scraped along somewhere in their deepest subconscious. They couldn't tolerate the banality of the biographies they were constantly correcting. Instead, and with Daddy's financial support, they exchanged texts about his various misdemeanours and discussed them to death until their own void felt confused and interesting again. They tore open diverse chasms so their cries would resonate. But there was nothing there.

They had no problems, but they took them very seriously.

For a long time, I'd been the exact opposite.

34

There was no solution, nothing to hold on to. Dying was only being postponed. The first of May came around, traditionally a local Kreuzberg mini-revolution that now also featured a street festival. I went and felt completely isolated among all those people, trapped in the notion of inhabiting a space that was different from theirs. I had nothing to do with them and they had nothing to do with me. I bit into a steak on a bun, then had to throw it away. Some kind of music blared off the stages. Lifeless bustle. Years ago, we'd had champagne, Bianca, Knut, Aljoscha and I, and felt a glamorous part of the revolutionary folklore. Now it was just a dead carnival. I went home and I knew: that was it.

Let the Cat Out of the Bag, a film with Jule Böwe, who I now knew, was still showing. I'd already seen it, but I let it run, wanted to have another look at Jule's breasts, masturbated unsuccessfully, and then took the pills. Way over two hundred, one after the other. Maybe I would just not wake up again.

When I did wake up the next day, in tremendous pain and with a full-body nausea I couldn't understand, I convinced myself to just stay put and wait it out until my liver was finished. But that turned out to be difficult. I stuck it out till noon, till early afternoon. The situation was no longer tenable. I couldn't even move. A painful pulsing and every nerve seemed to be nauseated. Every pore of my body wanted to puke. I called emergency services, stammering that I wasn't feeling good, I'd just tried to commit suicide. Clearly an appellative attempt, I realize today. And absolutely ridiculous. But I happen not to be a hero. What is that anyway, a "hero"?

The man on the line told me to take a taxi to the hospital. Which was wonderfully grotesque. I packed a few things into a bag and tried to set off. The Urban Hospital wasn't far. But after ten steps I couldn't go on; I was choking. I actually called a taxi, I must have had just enough money.

In emergency they gave me activated charcoal that I immediately puked up with a loud roar. Then they hooked me up to a drip, and infused an antidote. It seemed a liver transplant might be necessary, and I was moved to intensive care in another hospital. I wasn't told about the possible liver transplant and said nothing, asked nothing, let it all happen, and was hardly present. I came to on the third floor of the new hospital, in a room whose windows weren't locked, which struck me as ironic while offering me a last chance to get unironically serious. But I didn't jump. I didn't want to inflict that on the quiet older gentleman in the other bed. There are always excuses.

I wanted Aljoscha to come, and he came. I phoned my editor, whose familiar voice was comforting. Within a couple of hours I developed a rash on my chest. My liver was already recovering, I was told. A half litre of vodka on top, they said, would have finished it off. I had a very robust liver. My life was such a farce.

35

I spent months in the closed psych ward of the Urban Hospital. I participated in everything and felt I could trust some of the doctors. They, in their turn, pumped me full of medication, which I swallowed without resistance. Shared a room with a dim giant baby who kept uttering racist comments about the other patients and without my asking recommended the best places to masturbate. Endured that.

Frau Ulla Unseld-Berkéwicz offered support with a small Suhrkamp bursary. I need to mention this because later things came to a disastrous head between us, and I don't want to give the impression that it was her fault. But I do remember that these payments didn't kick in while I was in hospital because I was still collecting unemployment and welfare benefits at that point, as some job centre employee later painstakingly spelled out for me. Because, he said, anyone who is in hospital gets enough to eat, which is why I was expected to pay back a large part of the support, a certain number of per diems, overnight money for the weeks I was there, and I-don't-know-what-all. It was not helpful.

The kiosk only sold Coke, no newspapers. And usually not even Coke. Maybe gumdrop-like things, and always cigarettes. Dirk von Lowtzow appeared on the cover of the *Stadtmagazin*, and I felt no connection even though I'd published a review of the last Tocotronic album in *Freitag*. Fandom is exclusionary and once it's been destroyed can hardly be reconstructed later. Instead, the fallen pop star Joachim Deutschland landed in the next ward.

And so did Şenol, the son of my local convenience store owner from across the street, who was an actor in both RTL-TV and indie films. We had quite a few conversations on the ward, although once released we pretended to hardly know each other. These subterfuges are not healthy, and Şenol would probably have a few more things to say about all that, for other reasons. Unfortunately, he can't anymore, he killed himself later.

A three-bed room. Played chess regularly with a paranoid schizophrenic, an awkward, kind-hearted lawyer. The internet had driven him crazy, too. If I said I'd been on his homepage, he'd twitch even though he'd given me the address himself the day before. The viruses that he suspected were in the web had invaded his thoughts. But I think he's recovered and managed to stabilize himself. He was not a hopeless case.

Quite the contrast with about one-third of the patients. The so-called "revolving door patients" were noisily present. People who couldn't get free of their illness and came back every few months, whose lives had completely deteriorated with the hardships these attacks caused. Noses burst open, skin distended, logical thinking largely destroyed. It makes my heart ache, looking back. But at that time I was practically one of them.

And so memory wears thin in the daily grind. Your perception is muffled, your head, which is already slow as a result of the depression, is taken into chemical custody by mood modifiers, SSRIs and antidepressants. I and another patient were reduced to expressing thanks to the nurse for letting us finish watching the game show *Schlag den Raab* (Beat the Raab). Breakfast (the little bun was the highlight of the day), smoking room, ten minutes of some kind of exercise. When I tried a couple of dunks with a soft Pilates ball into a basketball net in the little gym rather than do rhythmic gymnastics with a club or a ball or a stretchy band, the pain was intense. Once upon a time, in my school days, I'd been a basketball player, but that had never been as far away as it was now.

At some point my agent Robert picked me up and took me back to my apartment. The neighbours, Karl-Uwe, an old Kreuzberg activist, who lived a few floors above me, and Petra, the artist who lived across the landing, were shocked when they saw me in the courtyard, at first for fear of some new terror I might set off, and then for the sense of destruction I emanated.

I participated in everything, clueless, but alive. Even attended the day clinic for weeks. One of the doctors I liked had been transferred there, someone who liked people, spoke with a clear voice, and treated his patients with just the right blend of humanity and distance. The sun shone down from above and had nothing to do with us. Something was going on all the time: pottery, crocheting, sculpting, although I tried to avoid all that and preferred sketching. But I went. A manic woman insisted on getting everybody to watch *Momo* with her. I sighed and joined in. *Michael Ende, only you are to blame—*

Gradually I started working again. After *Europe Central* was set aside (and ended up defeating a number of translators before it became a glorious success a few years later), I was offered *Riding Toward Everywhere,* also by William T. Vollmann, as a make-work project. In the last days of my manic bout, Yvonne had encouraged me to apply for a stay at an artists' residence at Künstlerdorf Schöppingen, where she was applying, and which I'd never heard of. Oddly enough, I was accepted, and she wasn't. Now I didn't know what to do. It didn't really matter, so I went.

36

Train stations, shopping spaces bathed in cold light, goods inside them shrink-wrapped in plastic, orders to buy, product alienation, just-in-time labour. Waiting on platforms, what for? Supposedly trains. You're a ghost but you feel the weight of your body, so you can't be a ghost, but what are you? Unwelcoming places, pressed into in-between spaces and seats, besieged by an unforgiving grief that will stay, between the places that are all without meaning, a book in your pocket that resists being read because your head is closed off, insulated from the world.

37

At the artists' residence, a sleepy, unspectacular house with a few outlying apartments, I maintained a sort of routine, partly involved in the social life: barbecuing and chatting, a bit of drinking. The days dribbled by, monotonous and see-through, into the void. One walk through the wheat fields, and then no more. Grit your teeth, eat, eat some more, don't think too much, go for walks, stay in bed, go to the supermarket across the way, stay in bed, avoid the supermarket across the way.

Supermarket, supermarket, supermarket. I could actually describe my entire life in terms of the supermarkets I've frequented, and my hatred of them, a hatred that has particular nuances that attach to each individual supermarket, the particular phase of my life and the qualities of the franchise itself. The frustrations, the despair, the heights of joy, the indifference that surfaced in that ever-similar lighting, or didn't, my view of that useless but still somehow necessary stuff in the shopping cart I continued to drag across the sticky floor just as I dragged the useless but somehow necessary content of my thoughts through my sticky consciousness; the shopping carts, the light that seemed to be coming through yellow-tinted glass. Pizzas over there, laundry soap there, and most of it I didn't even register. Doesn't matter if you're in an up-market shopping paradise or some rancid discount place—it's always the same humiliation. As long as I've been shopping I have hated shopping. I always feel out of place and have to leave as fast as I can.

So avoid the supermarket and stay in bed. Shovel in cornflakes. Want to die.

The reverberating shock that I had gone crazy again in the last year, and had lost everything inside and out, was lodged in my bones. And around these bones, due to an addiction to chocolate, grew a layer of fat, adhering to the old shapes like lint. Such a sluggish vegetative state.

Only chatting was possible, with Phoebe in England, for instance. Occasional conversations in the evening, strange and alien as always: all of them.

One night I received a call from my distraught mother. She wanted to kill herself, on the spot. My aunts were having her committed.

I wondered, what more?

38

And I only partially recovered. While I'd been able to recover completely in the years after 1999 and lead a life that was open to the future and full of possibilities, a life that allowed for real relationships and completely restored my soul and my mood, leaving only a few scrapes and fright at the adolescent abyss—the feeling of basically having been destroyed remained this time. I couldn't get rid of it. It was impossible to fill the cracks. The shards no longer fit together. But still I gathered new, damaged courage, new strength, as a form of resistance—resistance against my own fate—as existential defiance: let's see if a failure like me doesn't also have the right to exist.

It was quiet in my apartment at the residence. I worked, thought about new manuscripts, watched Alfred Hitchcock's early work on my laptop, having unwittingly bought it in my manic moments without really knowing why. Read Daniel Kehlmann and Thomas Glavinic, without much benefit.

I participated in a writing workshop at the Düsseldorf Schauspielhaus theatre, with a set of young, semi-depressed playwrights, and enjoyed the bright, lightning-quick personality of Thomas Jonigk, the seminar leader. A successful life was, apparently, possible. But no usable drama materialized, only three and a half attempts and a flat, short text.

The Theaterhaus in Jena offered me a writing contract to develop another play. I agreed. I became part of a theatre group I enjoyed there. My mood lightened, nothing went wrong. The play turned out okay, a Frankenstein rewrite. Then I dramatized a sci-fi novel that taught me a lot about form. Work helped.

And then back to Berlin, where the dumbos go when they can't think of anything else to do. I stuck it out in the apartment at Kottbusser Tor, which struck me as a shabby hotel room, but I felt relatively good in Kreuzberg, a sort of second home full of freaks and people who'd flipped out, all survivors of something. I still made big detours around certain bars. Tourists were slowly starting to take over.

The days were either filled with new work, or depending, with nothing. I opted for work. I still drank myself into oblivion in the city's bars, sometimes into a semi-manic delirium that caused an all-the-more merciless existential hangover the next day that was hard to endure. But I wanted to forget, and what else could I do for fun in this world that had turned so cold? Even without the illness it had been hard to take.

To cite a fellow sufferer, namely Edgar Allan Poe: "But I am constitutionally sensitive—nervous in a very unusual degree. I became insane, with long intervals of horrible sanity. During these fits of absolute unconsciousness I drank, God only knows how often or how much. As a matter of course, my enemies referred the insanity to the drink rather than the drink to the insanity." So are you just getting drunk, or are you already manic? Are you drinking because you are sick, or are you sick because you drink?

I won two awards for *Raumforderung*, my short story collection, which surprised and pleased me, even though the accompanying events were more modest, cooler and

less spectacular than I'd once imagined. I was only barely able to produce the acceptance speech for the Bremen
literature prize. What was I supposed to say? "If you have
a problem with something, make that the topic," Jonigk
advised. So that's what I did. That's what I'm doing now.
I was not yet subject to panic attacks during speeches or
readings at that point and so I got through without incident,
before an audience of venerable seniors and schoolchil-
dren condemned to attend the ceremony. At the dinner at
city hall afterward I sat next to the journalist Lothar Müller,
who told interesting stories about Botho Strauss and the
United States. I, on the other hand, kept quiet, like a frightened child.

Outside city hall, a crazy lady started jabbering at me.
The shadows on our faces merged.

The meaning of all this remained inaccessible to me. But
at least I was able to keep going.

39

2008, 2009: shot at and injured, but not down. A summer
that, here and there, began to feel like summer again. Evenings on the canal, away from everyone but still present.
Fixed up the apartment a little. My mother recovered. I kept
fiddling around with *Sickster*. Observed people in the cafés
and wondered what they were doing there. Did my rounds,
still filled with shame. Read a lot again. Even though no
actual form became visible, bits of content remained.

The disappointment and alienation from yourself, the
burden of having thought and perpetrated so much nonsense, the cancellation of most of the plans for your life,
persevering against all that, getting up in the morning,
reaching new objectives, and still the loss of a general
meaning to life, and of a goal-oriented biography, if there

even is such a thing. Deep gashes in your chest, boundless disillusionment. Getting up in the morning, over and over again, against gravity, against the need to just stay there forever, still goes on. Only three cups of coffee, then later a slight fever, then the hectic rush—the emotional lows and highs are still there, the ups and downs typical of the illness still come on, but much less vehement. Creating a structure for yourself, even if it's seldom respected; seeking to lose yourself in your work, the moment in pianists' performances when they merge with others. But structure has its dangers too: when it turns into stress, when bureaucratic duty becomes a depressing malaise; and you can't sleep too much either, otherwise that depressed mood will show up again and your warding it off can trigger a manic attack. But then, if you don't sleep enough, mania is an imminent threat. *Oh boy.*

Mixing with others is a duty you perform. Losing yourself in conversation. Thinking pragmatically and somehow taking part in what's going on outside. Sometimes feeling that maybe things don't have to be quite as bad as they seem.

40

It was idiotic, but I stopped taking the pills. I didn't want to keep on taking them forever. I didn't think the madness could so soon take possession of me again, I was still far too destroyed from the last episode. How could the system muster the strength to boot up again and attack? As an organism I was too idle, too fat, and too weak, paralyzed by the medication and bloating into a shapeless mass, just like my thinking.

It is not easy to accept that you will have to be on medication for life. And the doctors don't tell you that with the necessary emphasis either. But it is plainly the case: bipolar disorder is an illness that returns, often with serious and fatal consequences, and so the treatment is not just momentary; it is a lifelong therapy supported by medication. But that is hard to take in, especially when you already feel like you're just a bundle of side effects. The younger you are, the more you refuse to believe.

I quietly dropped the medication, the Orfiril, an anticonvulsant with a phase-stabilizing effect, as well as the serotonin reuptake inhibitor. *Brain zaps*, small electric shocks in my head and body were the result. Since then, the effects of dropping the serotonin reuptake inhibitor have been recognized and described. At the time, this was not the case, and when I told doctors about the shocks they stared in disbelief. A pharmacologist friend did the research and discovered that brain zaps are, in fact, known but had not been included in the official catalogue of side effects—the lobby, the lies, the money. They disappear after two or three weeks and are not dangerous. But besides the very unpleasant sensation of an electric shock in the brain that beams into every part of you, they cause serious irritation. Have I lost all control of myself? Is this nothing but a neurochemical game of chance? What is going on? Electric shocks from within!

I waited, without really realizing it. I endured.

Around me, people were setting up middle-class lives. I believe this is called marriage. It comprised children, a structure, and a future. I didn't even have a present.

41

Just now, as I was writing about "middle-class lives," I briefly thought about differences in habitus and wanted to reach for Pierre Bourdieu's *Distinction* to read a little. It was just half a thought, a preconscious wish. It couldn't be fulfilled. Because there was nothing to reach for. There's nothing left. I'd had three or four books by Bourdieu in my collection; all of them are gone. When I see the cover of a book I once owned, like Bob Dylan's *Chronicles* yesterday, I feel a small stab of pain. When I come across a copy of a book I once owned, I know it immediately. I have a passive memory of all the books I ever owned. It never stops.

42

Over Christmas Aljoscha and I flew to Turkey, to Istanbul. We moved into our room in the Grand Hotel de Londres that served as a location for the film *Head-On,* and discovered the city. Istanbul was much more hectic and crowded than I'd expected, a real metropolis, suspended between the centuries—as we were suspended between the years—and was neither of today nor of yesterday, but rather of both. We roamed through Beyoğlu, drank Efes, checked out the student scene, ate fish on Galata Bridge and looked at sabres in the Topkapı Palace. Only on the ferries did we realize how busy Istanbul actually was, and it seemed that only there could these bustling people ever come to rest and breathe deeply. Those were lovely days.

On the flight home I was so wrecked from the night before that a passenger sitting next to Aljoscha asked him what was wrong with his friend. Nothing, I said, nothing at all. What could possibly be wrong?

On New Year's Eve I got lost, snow everywhere, I couldn't find my friends, though I was pretty familiar with the area around the Helmholtzplatz where the party was taking place. I was too impatient to hang around for a taxi. I headed out, my cell phone had no connection, and I fell into the wet snow.

The future was open, with limitations, I thought on New Year's Day, as I finished writing the last lines of a new drama for Jena, *The Heart Is a Lousy Hustler*. It had turned into a melodramatic comedy: on the one hand, like Ingrid Lausund's play *Tür auf, Tür zu* (Door Open, Door Shut), and on the other hand, breathy nicotine-ridden pathos in a green evening gown. I was getting new ideas.

I didn't know that these ideas would be abruptly cut back and shredded by the destructive mechanisms of mania—as silly as they are deadly. I knew so little. The days drifted across the land and through me. Maybe there was a countdown hanging over me. I managed to meet Aljoscha and Knut in the Alt Berlin bar, and they later commented (which is always easy to do) that I had already seemed "different" that evening. My new blog, which I hadn't stopped talking about, was given some of the blame. I cannot confirm or deny any of that. But something was brewing, and I was actually provoking it—by writing the blog and discontinuing the medication.

God was lying in wait. The disaster was lying in wait.

2010

1

Uh-huh, him

—until a voice timidly arose again from the sea of whispering, rustling, ticking, peeping sounds, still rather fragile, a first throat-clearing, sound check, one two, one two, yeah, yeah, yeah, the system seems to be working, that's a start, so shall we begin? Are we ready to go? But where? The marionettes nodded in silence: *go ahead, say something.* I'm sure I've been here before, I hummed, but where exactly wasn't very clear, I thought, every syllable a step in swampy territory while beyond the line of trees over there the first firecrackers of the New Year were banging away, lit by young Turks who'd hoarded them churlishly and who thought this was just the right moment to trigger them into snowmashed explosions.

And this is meant to go on till the day of the publication?
And you, you in particular, you dare get back into the internet?
You know perfectly well, that you—how should I say this—no?
But otherwise you're fine?

Meanwhile a first pressure in my head and a cryptic gentle easing of my shortness of breath. Oh, the affectation will give way too, after it's raised a little stink over the course of a couple of entries, I reassured myself, in confusion: and the urge to say everything at once too. Welcome back to the *Sickster*, my fingers said, a blog on my book at the time of its creation, with all weaknesses and flaws included, inclined toward everything grand and gross. You've never been here before? Don't get too comfortable. It makes you like to control your tone of voice because it sounds wrong, not yours, too cultivated, even blasé; it wrongly assigns a particular wrong space to what is not your own. But there's plenty of room, isn't there, I thought, there is so much room available, no worries, young man, simply get started, *feel free to feel free and feel weird*, and go ahead, let the illness slowly reclaim its right to speak; let what silenced you become audible.

My time will come in 2010—if we meet again; the conditional aspect of this "if" that earlier was only thinkable as highly exclusive and quite unreal, internally a completely mad unreal-unreality, luckily changed to a very feasible temporal form—*when we meet*— just like that, over time. In the end everything will be there, properly calibrated and balanced, in the end enough words will have been uttered, enough reflections pumped out, in the end, at some point; small, virus-like particles, all electric again, supporting or cancelling each other out in friction and tension, usually both, will finally have been written out and congealed as the novel about my life, unfortunately, and this blog along with all its functions, the actual ones as well as the imaginary ones, will be gone; and then we'll see, see the horizon, and move on into the realm of fictions, finally, finally. *We'll*

jus' see, and then we'll see, is what the kaiser dictated to
the pageboys in his narcissism and relaxedness, and
of course in cursive script, exactly that, totally cursive,
ladies and gentlemen, cursivecursivecursive, *exacto-
mundo,* the standpipe's dry, he added quickly, already
bald and weak, because of Wittgenstein, the fly in the
glass and the standpipe-typical nature of those functions that were already destined to disappear; for what
goes up will quickly be shot down; and the fool, still
innocent and curly haired, listened up and sharpened
his pencil. Body scanners came zooming up. The joyful
melancholy of a beginning came blowing through an
apartment called a "hole."

(My first blog post, January 1, 2010)

2

We were sitting in a restaurant called Kuchenkaiser: the
dramaturge, the director, the set designer, and me. I must
have been pretty much out of reach. Something was fes-
tering in me again.

Still, I made an attempt to join the discussion, take part
in a conversation, keep an open mind, and kept running
into opposition. Two fronts had formed before I even got
there, and those fronts were dramaturgy and text versus
direction and set design. The director and the set designer apparently opposed the text, they didn't like it, but they
didn't know why. Or they didn't want to say. Or they liked
it, but had decided to oppose it anyhow. Or they just didn't
know, had no real position, and as a precaution were closing
themselves off, stupidly aloof. They sat there across from
me, pretty remote, and exuded a jittery kind of arrogance
that got on my nerves since it had no purpose or direction.

The set designer, whom I knew slightly, had cut off his heavy-metal-style ponytail and was now sporting a funky undercut hairdo. It all seemed like something out of a neon-radiated new wave pub of the 1980s where self-conscious provincials test out their big-city look. Except that we were in the early years of the twenty-first century, in Kreuzberg, in a rather stuffy restaurant, and were supposed to be discussing how to make a new text work. It was bizarre.

In the theatre, such fronts are drawn every day. Directors consider authors their natural enemies, and authors see directors as a necessary evil. It was nothing special, just the daily vanities of the struggles that take place in the orchestra pit; these two were just overdoing it a bit. The dramaturge later let off some steam about the two "junior artists." I grinned, relieved that I was not alone in my assessment of their behaviour.

And yet there was a sensitivity in me. I felt particularly put out by their posturing and I registered their little vanities differently than I would have otherwise. Their inhibited gestures sent overly strong signals, and their blasé expressions were a direct affront. The absurdities were so impressive. I tried to find reasons for their attitude. It couldn't just have to do with the play, could it? That would be silly. An idea came to me: had they maybe read my blog and got scared?

3

In December, I'd fiddled around with programming the blog, if you can call it that. At least I'd spent days working on the source code, changed the colours of the template, deleted visual effects in the html mode I didn't like, all that—learning by doing. It was supposed to go online on New Year's Day, and that's what happened, accompanied

by a Nine Inch Nails live video of "Somewhat Damaged."
Reznor performed a powerful clockwise gesture with his
left arm; so, the clock had struck twelve. I sent an email
to friends, acquaintances, and so-called influencers and
began happily typing away. The blog was going to be a running commentary on the novel *Sickster* that I had taken up
again to force myself to keep working every day, it would
be a work in progress, a diary of my writing project, exploring the difficult relationship between autobiography and
fiction. And it was meant to simply narrate what it's like
to live with bipolarity. It was supposed to be a start on this
current book and at the same time inspire and reflect on
the work for another book, as well as being a normal blog,
of the kind other people evidently enjoyed producing. Lots
of stuff for one page.

I didn't think I was in any danger. But I should have
realized that immediate, unedited online publications had
once already been the trap door to my illness. I wanted
to work, wanted to let rip, saw that systematic and speedy
writing was the solution to stasis, to life sluggishly slipping
by. My friends were skeptical.

The project started to keel over with the very first entries.
I spent time finessing the texts and didn't deal with the
book, spent hours pondering which music videos I should
use as accompaniment, wrote things that were already a
touch too intimate. Suddenly my *Sickster* protagonist was
a filmmaker who was meant to spew out his hatred, actually my hatred, for the so-called Berlin School. I wrote
about apologies not doing much good because people still
didn't believe that a madman could ever be a person again;
they preferred to silence it all to death and laugh in horror
behind the guilty person's back. I wrote something about
my grandfather, a heavy scene from my childhood, where

he'd washed his penis in the kitchen, and grinned at me while he was doing it. Agitated, I put it all online. Today, I think my grandfather's grinning was not even so terrible, but the fired-up condition I was in turned the memory of such things into monstrosities. I had already lost myself.

Then I woke up one morning, it must have been around January 10. I have already written an alienated, altered, shortened version of the scene in *3000 Euros*.

4

Back to the relationship between me and my characters. So far, my protagonists have all been versions of myself, all sharing the same basic constitution, the same basic destiny, but equipped with certain new characteristics that turn them into autonomous figures who can operate on their own. Some of the details in my fictional texts relate directly to my life, many do not. I think writing like this is quite a common practice.

But I don't want to keep stewing in my own juice. Which is why this book is an attempt to write myself free of this eternal revenge. Because if I don't write myself free, I will remain stuck, I know, and my writing will continue to be populated and weighed down by these doppelgängers, who in the end keep referring back to me, laying me bare and at the same time concealing me.

Saying "I" under these circumstances is not at all easy, and I do so with all the more determination. If I don't try to round up my stories, fetch them back, raise my voice on my own account without faking it, I will remain a zombie in my life, especially in my life, a version of myself, just like my characters.

At the same time, I am, of course, writing myself ever further offside, further than I already am. I'll end up as the "manic-depressive," alone, over there in the corner. All the better: it'll give me something I can write against.

And in fact, it is also the exact opposite: I have been standing in that corner for years and only now am I abandoning it.

5

So it must have been around the tenth of January. I woke up in a panic. My brain was pressing against my skull. I clutched my head. My arms and legs were tingling. What was this? There was nausea in my head. I leaped up, still in panic. Where should I go? There was too much energy. I couldn't say more. I couldn't say anything, I was wordless. I didn't know what to do with all the bad energy pulsing through me. I plunged around the room, out of all control, agitated, whatever was wrong? Spent a long blank moment in front of my crowded clothes rack. There was no longer a point of conjunction called "I." There were only qualia: sensations clustered around animalistic instinct, and God.

God? I looked over to the window and out into the grey sky. He looked back. There was God. But which God? What? I felt him, *it*, its gaze. The sky was really staring at me. Holy shit: God. I felt sick.

6

I had lost God when I optimized prayer. Since my earliest childhood I had recited two long standard prayers every evening, at an irritating and masochistically slow pace so that I wouldn't be berated for rushing through them or being superficial. Between the two prayers, I'd always had a rather lengthy conversation with God that was a recapitulation of the day and a wish list for the next day and the near future. These conversations were the central core of the ritual in the dark, and the two standard prayers were the frame. Sometime around the age of eleven or twelve, the prayers started being rattled off more and more quickly and the dialogue was reduced to the essentials, soon working with repetitions and blocks of phrases. I was optimizing my prayers, in terms of time spent and format used. Pragmatism moved into my childhood bed. The framing prayers were churned out ever more quickly and the actual conversation was hardly thought through. The sign of the cross consisted of a brief tap of fingers on my chest. Once the whole thing had degenerated into a sloppily rapped-out blur of language, I abandoned the prayer ritual. Which also caused God to die. That was a shock but there was no way back. When I lost my line to the highest authority, I also lost my belief in its existence. And when a gaunt old priest who reminded me of Harry Kane, the reverend in *Poltergeist II*—I remember that exactly—when he asked me at confession if masturbation was already an issue for me, I was also finished with the institution. I didn't go to confession again, I refused the imminent confirmation. I also dropped communion during the obligatory masses that were held at school. I didn't like it, but I was now an atheist. And I could sense that when the form falls apart, so does the content.

7

But now I was the one falling apart. For entire minutes my existence was extinguished. And yet, outside, in the gleaming grey, there was still this energy, stronger than me, in the air, in the atmosphere, in the breadth of the sky. I was connected to it, I was *meant*, in a strange, all-encompassing way I was meant from the outside, recognized by the universe, singled out, seized. Even in dissolution it found me, and took me up, but it was hostile. There was nothing concrete about all this, there were no explanations that might have pointed to an outer reality or causes and connections. It was not yet paranoia or psychosis, only a shift into pure form. Something had entered me full force, something without a valve, boiling hot until the boundaries of the ego melted away. The madness was still without an owner, still unbound, it stood there alone, naked, blank, without concepts.

I felt nauseous again, not as though I needed to vomit, but over my entire body, *throughout* my entire body. I didn't know what to do with myself; go here, go there, it was all going wrong. A pressure inside me was hammering outward in all directions. My breath and heart were racing. A mash of ideas was brewing in my head. What was that on my foot? I must have already been walking a lot. Who'd been walking? Me? Early memories and ideas came back. Me! Me and my foot. I was still wearing my socks. From yesterday? Yesterday! Yes, yesterday, that existed, there had been another day. One day? Days! They existed. I spun around and looked out the window again. Was God still out there?

A cramp developed in my calf when I focused my attention on it. Psychosomatic evidence for God, I thought. Yes: God had entered my consciousness as an enemy. And now I was godlike, too, got a cramp as soon as I imagined one in exactly the place where my perception indicated. I threw my body onto the mattress.

Lay there, beyond myself for a long time. But slowly an identity began to build again around these feelings, holding them loosely together. It wasn't the "I" of yesterday evening or the "I" of a week ago that was coming together here, already tangling, intertwining with falsehoods. But

"I" was "here." Hadn't that been the thesis of one of my former lecturers, his cogito, on which an entire theory of perception might be constructed: *I am here?* Had he passed it on to me as a ghostly incantation, or what? As a supplication, maybe, in case I ever had to deal with the consciousness of being reduced to absolute zero?

Gone again, that thought. But I did seem to have a past. There had been that lecturer Soldati, and there'd been this "I am here." That was years ago. So I'd already been around for years. That let me hold it together for a moment. But the cramp was still there, growing sharper. I'd forgotten that all I had to do was stretch my calf to get rid of the cramp. Then I remembered, but I tightened my calf instead. The pain grew hotter. I couldn't defend myself or move. Finally, the cramp receded.

I lay there and lay there. Then the panic returned. Something was wrong, that was clear. I had some kind of illness, something very acute. If I didn't call emergency now, I would never forgive myself. I would probably end up crippled for life. My leg might fall off. God would stay in my body as an enemy. I reached for the phone and dialed.

Waiting for the emergency doctor, I calmed down a little, felt like retracting the call. When the paramedics showed up, no doctor but mighty, bearded men, I hardly knew what to tell them. But I was still panicky. They examined my leg and found nothing. But this here, they said, this must be athlete's foot.

Was that supposed to be a joke? And if so, on whose part?

They huddled over me and looked at me skeptically, apathetic, swelled-up faces behind scruffy beards. My voice was trembly as I apologized. I didn't know what was wrong, I sang hoarsely: I guess I've gotten into a bit of a panic.

Then they left.

They probably figured drugs were involved. Maybe they laughed or grumbled on the way back.

I lay there, I just lay still, and slowly the well-known old messiah paranoia crept over my thinking, but it was grubbier this time, more washed-out, less defined than it had been earlier, without the iridescent exactitude it had before; it was more of a raw, recurring, general impulse. The paranoia was fraying and threadbare like an old worn-out glove that you pull on and hardly feel on your skin.

I jumped up, slid on my shoes, and stormed out of the apartment.

And God was forgotten.

8

The events of this year can be partially reconstructed with reference to the cultural functions I participated in. There was the premiere of a play by René Pollesch. I have to check back when exactly that was: January 12, 2010. We'd made a date. I was out in front of the Volksbühne Theatre with Patrick, feeling agitated. I'm not sure how bizarre the impression I was making may have been, perhaps I was still able to fake ordinary small talk. It was late, we were waiting for Aljoscha. Christoph Schlingensief, terminally ill, drove up in a taxi, got out, walked up the steps, looked at us, his face lighting up, and gave us a nod.

"How friendly," Patrick said, "I don't even know him."

But I did. We'd known each other for a long time, or so I thought, ever since 1999. And of course, went my thoughts, scraping up the sediment of my subconscious, it was because of me that Schlingensief had lost it and fallen ill.

Because I, too, was sick. My internal search for why I was suddenly feeling so unwell had generated the self-diagnosis of AIDS. I had AIDS, I was sure of it, the disease whose existence I had once refuted in 1999. I figured that I'd probably contracted the virus in Turkey and I imagined that I'd been deliberately infected. Aljoscha hadn't taken good enough care of me, in fact he'd literally delivered me up to the source of the virus, a Turkish student. That was my off-the-cuff diagnosis. And so the rage that was gathering in me had a reason and a purpose.

Aljoscha came running up the steps, and we went in.

We had to make do with beanbags for seating, and I couldn't get comfortable, couldn't find the right position, before the play even started. A woman I didn't know ended up pressing me into the beanbag, which oddly enough calmed me down. It was a moment that made everyone laugh.

I wasn't at all interested in what was going on onstage. The stunts of Fabian Hinrichs, the actor, left me cold. I found certain phrases irritating, they either had too much or nothing to do with me. I couldn't sit still, and after about twenty minutes I left the performance, slamming the door. It was historic, Aljoscha said sarcastically afterward. Or was he sarcastic? It was getting harder and harder to recognize irony.

I wandered around, had a beer somewhere, waited outside for the end of the premiere, turned up at the party. I talked and talked at Aljoscha, that the AIDS diagnosis was real, that I felt panicky. Aljoscha set aside his usual scorn and tried to reassure me about how slight the chances of such an infection were. He couldn't get through to me. I went over to Schorsch Kamerun and confessed that I'd uploaded a song by his band Goldene Zitronen on my blog. Kamerun said it was too late now anyway, I should have asked permission earlier. I bounced back and forth, and Patrick and Aljoscha decided to take me to the Prassnik

Bar so we could talk. When we got to this bar, with its phony Eastern bloc ambience, I worked myself up even more into my AIDS panic, and added the feeling of having-been-betrayed for years. Once again, those closest to me were those farthest away; they'd deliberately kept me uninformed and thereby diminished me. Rage washed over me in waves, I alternated between silence and shouting in anger, prophesying, "I'm going to get skinnier now." At some point Patrick disappeared, which left Aljoscha trying to talk sense into me. I got even angrier. Then I reined myself in and tried to stay calm. No chance.

Finally, out in the street, I punched Aljoscha, hitting him so hard that he landed flat out in the street. I'd crossed a boundary. I'd often had bouts of aggression, but they'd never turned into physical attacks on friends. Now it had happened. My friendship with Aljoscha was never the same after this. And that was just the beginning of the breakdown that was to follow. I saw him as a traitor who'd never told me what was really going on. He saw me as a madman who could no longer be trusted, and who attacked his own friends. I was wrong, he was right. Two solitudes began to take shape.

9

But a manic doesn't feel lonely, even if he is lonely in an absolute, quite unimaginable way. At least in my head I was in constant dialogue with everything and everyone. These dialogues-in-my-head had always been part of my world. Everyone has their own experience of them: the anticipation, the hindsight, or the plain old invention of conversations that are not connected to real events—sometimes hotter, sometimes cooler than would ever be possible in reality, sometimes with the addition of a corrective final point. But I no longer had any control over these dialogues in my head; endlessly ongoing discussions rushed through my mind in wild tatters, unmanageable. And the culture was again broadcasting massively in my direction—the news too. I reacted in my blog and in online forums, talking to ghosts. But language kept slipping away from me. Right from the start, I was producing shreds of Dada that even I could hardly understand. And the grand overarching superstructure of paranoia reinstalled itself, yet hardly registered as a shock or a spectacle. It had become routine.

The premiere in Jena was coming up. I'd heard that the rehearsals had been difficult, that the director was making small cuts in the style and micro-structure of the script. This infuriated me. I can live with generous cuts at macro levels but I insist on the micro-details of my some-times rather overwritten style. There is a real contrastive difference between a character saying they want to hear "clichéd classical music," and just "classical music." The director didn't seem to have woken up to this point. And the manic had found the next deconstruction site for his crazed bulldozer.

Word apparently got back to Jena fast that the author of the play had gone crazy. Some of the actors wondered what such an illness might mean for the script they were sup-posed to perform, whether this script might now be some-how uncanny and crazy too. I can imagine that this might cause a reticence with regard to the words on the page. The portents had changed, the lines might be poisoned.

I headed off to Jena, unannounced, disrupted the rehears-als, once, twice, three times. The theatre folks didn't know how to handle me. Marvin, the theatre director, a good, easygoing guy, stayed calm and tried to smooth things over. I remember completely flipping out one evening in the kitchen of the apartment at the theatre. It had nothing to do with the play, I'd simply been seized by enormous grief and fear, and started yelling and weeping. The set designer yelled at me to shut up. Maybe a good response, maybe a different way to break the madness. The director stayed calm, the dramaturge had already fallen silent. I was in a total panic when I went off into the living room that was designated as mine, assuming they were planning to murder me. Joking, the director had said that in order to subdue that fear I should probably set something breakable in front of the door. In my confusion, I actually did that, then it seemed absurd and I put the glass back on the table. I heard them talking in the kitchen, helplessly debating what to do, I leaped up again, and leaning against the door frame, uttered some kind of nonsense. I said I couldn't possibly sleep there, I probably couldn't sleep at all, but there, in enemy territory, it was absolutely impossible.

They took me to a hotel that looked like a vicious brothel. I took a Tavor I still had from Aljoscha, and then fantasized that the tranquillizer was making me hallucinate. I saw patterns and images slide past my mind's eye. Meanwhile Tavor is anything but hallucinogenic. The question is whether imagined hallucinations aren't also real hallucinations. Anyway, I imagined that I would now die, that Aljoscha had quietly poisoned me.

I called emergency services, they came by and wanted to pick me up, I refused to go. The next morning Hauke, a director closely connected to the theatre, was alerted to take me back to a hospital in Berlin. I fled. People went looking for me. Someone had broken a window at the back of the theatre, they suspected me. Meanwhile I was tearing through the streets of Jena, thinking about the early Romantics, about Friedrich Schiller, feeling I had somehow travelled back into their era and was really living in the past, able to follow the thought processes of Johann Gottlieb Fichte more concretely than ever before: one spontaneous action, here within me, the ineluctable positing of the "I," and another spontaneous action, now, and another one. Somehow Marvin found me. He was one of the few people I believed I could still trust, but as I was getting into his car I noticed a cable running along the edge of the side window. It was probably just a normal radio cable. But wait a minute! Hadn't someone made a joke last night, while casting a sideways glance in my direction, that Marvin was with the police? So what kind of a cable was that? Certainly not a normal cable! More likely a direct connection to headquarters. Suddenly, and without any flash of recognition that this assumption was quite absurd, Marvin was no longer a director for me, he was a policeman. He'd always been a policeman, and the theatre and everything around it were nothing but camouflage for a double life, that many people knew about. Except me, of course.

I gave up. They had me. Marvin patiently delivered me to the psychiatric ward in Jena. I spent the night there. When you've been in psychiatric wards as often as I have, they are the most boring places on earth. Nothing happens there.

The next day I broke out again.

10

Cornelia recaptured me, I took off. Hauke recaptured me, I took off. Hauke recaptured me again and took me back to Berlin by train. I still didn't want to let them lock me up. All well-meaning persuasion was in vain.

I roamed around in the world, in time as well as in space. Studied the occasional "almanac," looked for dates, found them, forgot them again. Because it really didn't matter how long this thing had been going on, what was clear was *that* it was going on, and that was an unacceptable outrage the world was committing against me. But my agitation was growing blurry: while my potential for aggression was greater than before, I could no longer find targets in the past, there were just impulses in the present. I was a tourist lost in his own mania. It was no longer so clearly silhouetted, no longer so evidently edgy and on the surface; it was hunkered deep down, darker, meaner, more intractable.

Leipzig became a new attraction for me, and so I drifted around there, "making sure things were on the right track," I said in an ambiguous reference to right-wing activities there. Stopped in at a restaurant where I'd been with friends years earlier. Talked to the wait staff about the rapper Sido. Travelled back to Berlin. Spent two days with a band in Kreuzberg, heading straight from a bar to their apartment. Travelled back to Leipzig. Hung around at the train station.

11

"You won't remember but last time you were here you left after a few shots of Jägermeister, and started interfering in traffic, directing traffic, sort of. You dragged a sign out into the street and caused a jam. You're not getting anything more right now. We'll talk about later another time."

"Okay!"

"You're under observation. If there's another report, we'll have to find a caregiver to keep an eye on you."

"Okay!"

"You know what they should do with you? Send you to the gas chamber."

"Okay!"

"C'mon, come and get me."

"Okay!"

"You've been diagnosed as fulfilling two or three of the six criteria of the ICD-10 for progressing from alcohol abuse to alcohol addiction. A light increase in liver enzymes and lab results show a macrocytic anemia—further indication of your obviously ongoing high consumption of alcohol."

"Okay!"

"Somebody really ought to smash your face!"

"Why?"

"Oh, just like that. This 'n' that."

"Okay!"

12

I bought the ticket to London in Hamburg, on a whim, because I absolutely had to go to London, where pop culture was born, that was my next idée fixe. I'd never been there, how absurd. Berlin had become too small for me, banning orders had become routine, and the traffic would continue to flow in its awful cycles without me.

On the flight, in business class of course, I used my new credit card to buy some aftershave and an external hard drive, mainly because the stewardess had such a charming British accent. Three rows ahead of me was (the actual) Andrew Fletcher of Depeche Mode. I set up my CD bag which I'd just finished decorating with the smeared logos and names of countless bands, including the DM of Depeche Mode, in such a way that he'd have to see it if he turned around. And I would see to that, discreetly.

Then we all fell asleep, stunned by a loud bang that I thought came from breaking through the sound barrier. Had we really broken through? Because there was no counting on experience, and knowledge was unreliable. We were in a time capsule, on our way into space, and maybe the

pilot was so pleased about this random get-together that
he stepped down hard on the accelerator. I mumbled for-
mulas into orbit.

When I woke up, Andrew Fletcher was looking at me
thoughtfully. Maybe no other person since then has gazed
at me as thoughtfully and seriously as Andrew Fletcher of
Depeche Mode did on that flight to London.

I didn't say a word.

When we arrived, I grabbed a taxi, with Peter Gabriel
driving. Smoking was not allowed though. Where to, is
what he wanted to know. Downtown, I said, some hotel.
I hadn't booked anything. At some point he dropped me
off in front of an expensive-looking hotel complex and I
checked in. I immediately called Cornelia in Jena and
would do that three or four more times that night, phoning
myself into debt, as I discovered later at the reception desk.
Cornelia talked everything through with me and calmed
me down. Meanwhile I was looking around the hotel room,
large-scale reproductions and the finest linen wallpaper.
I hung up and headed out to three or four clubs, where
I danced like a dervish. Because if you've only just realized that the parties are meant for you, that you're always
included even if you're absent, that ecstasy, for instance,
is not really a drug but a kind of host the others share with
you as at communion, in memory of yourself and with the
appropriate feelings of joy as a reward—then you really
want to join the celebration, as excessively as possible to
make up for the limitations your insufficient awareness
imposed over the past years.

And that's what I did.

During the day I strolled around London as you would
through a school textbook. Trafalgar Square, Piccadilly
Circus, Speakers' Corner, Buckingham Palace—I felt as

though I was leafing through these sights, as though they were two-dimensional and I wasn't really standing there in front of them. At some point I checked out of the hotel, the bill was impressive, and went looking for another one. I lost sight of this plan though, had a couple of pints in front of a pub, Kurt Cobain, still alive, was grumpily sipping a beer next to me. Then I headed back out into the night, started talking with young people I thought I knew from Myspace, which I'd recently started using because Conrad Keely once told me about it, in healthy times, backstage after a Trail of Dead concert. Then I lost my new smartphone and my jacket. I tried to extract some money from an ATM but the machine wouldn't give me any. I tried again, and was briefly scared I'd forgotten the PIN number, which I then promptly did. The situation grew more acute.

Day broke, and I had to get hold of some money because it was three more days till my return flight. But that was harder than I thought. I stumbled through the speedy city, avoided getting run down countless times. When I asked a girl where I might find a Deutsche Bank, she suggested I go buy something in a shop, pay for it by credit card, and ask for cash back. I couldn't make that work though, I was already almost paralyzed: completely stupid and couldn't understand. I entered a bank and went up to the counter. The alcohol on my breath immediately gave me away to the teller as a "naughty boy"; she even flirted with me and kept saying what a bad boy I must have been. But strangely she couldn't accept the credit card. She told me to wait for her on a specific bench in Hyde Park and in two hours she'd help me out privately. That was probably more of a tactic to get rid of me than an actual offer. Once in Hyde Park I sat down somewhere and fell asleep. Tramps with Russian accents came up and said they wanted to help. I didn't believe them.

I stomped off, with a few pounds left in my pocket, and lay down somewhere else. I no longer knew where exactly I was in London.

The banks offered no hope. My card was completely useless.

Finally, I got on the bus to Heathrow, dodging the fare. I was so exhausted when I got there, I just sat down and dozed. Then I jolted out of my daze, suddenly aware of my situation. I was sitting in the airport in London with no money and three more days ahead of me. How strange! I thought. Where was Damon Albarn when you needed him?

I tried to change my ticket, which incurred an extra charge. I couldn't pay that extra charge. I hated my credit card for being rejected all over the place, what a useless, absurd piece of plastic. "That's a case for the manager," the woman at the counter kept repeating. But the manager couldn't be located and she got rid of me, mission unaccomplished. Should I maybe go to the German Embassy as an emergency case? I knew that was an option from having been stranded in Prague when I was younger. But my cell phone was gone, and I no longer had the strength to go anywhere in this city. I had lost all orientation. And I was hungry.

I was friends with two British women via my new Facebook account, who'd even visited me in Berlin. I rummaged around for my last pence, found an internet terminal, logged on to Facebook and sent a cry for help to one of them, Phoebe, who was a student in London. She needed to lend me the money for a return flight, it was really an emergency, and no joke, I insisted. Then I logged off again, roamed through the airport, bummed some cigarettes. Two hours later I logged on again. No answer. I had just enough money to log on one more time. I counted the minutes, I was hungry, I tried to kill time somehow. Two hours later, one last log in. Phoebe had responded and was even online. She wrote that she'd be there in three hours. I told her at which entrance to meet and noted that on the palm of my hand.

When she finally came through the entrance and into the airport, she looked like a queen to me. And that's what she was. The automatic door opened up triumphantly, and against the light her silhouette appeared like an epiphany. I could hardly believe my luck. We joined the queue at the airline counter, chatting and joking. Why hadn't I got hold of Ruby, Phoebe asked, she'd have loved to show me around London. True, why hadn't I, I wondered. Phoebe gave no sign that she noticed how strange all this was, or how strange I was. Maybe the strangeness was even a little British? Finally, it was my turn and I asked for the next flight. It worked. When the price appeared on the screen, Phoebe simply smiled and said, "My treat."

We got something to eat and Phoebe made sure I didn't miss my flight. She was incredible. A few days later I sent her the money and thanked her effusively.

Looking back, I feel like I've never been in London.

13

"Do you know a Merle? Do you know a Merle? Are you related to her? That's good, too good, haha. Pretty soon you'll be in for it too!" The messages in the pop songs now revealed themselves to me in their full depth. The harder I listened, the more I of course gleaned. And I listened obsessively, on the go with earphones plugged in, my earphones were always new because the wear and tear was enormous. My jerky movements would rip off the cables. It was only because her first name sounded like my last name that a certain schoolgirl by the name of Merle was murdered in the 1980s, and the telephone terror that ensued and that the grieving family suffered was made public by the police to help find the perpetrator. The Einstürzende Neubauten used some of this material in their song "Die Elektrik (Merle)." And of course the Neubauten had phoned me anonymously and then integrated my unsteady "Hello," that was not yet quite sure of its sonority after my adolescent change of voice, in their song "Ich Bin's" (It's Me). It all fit exactly with the release dates.

Since everything was about me, I was part of everything, I kept getting messages I could either accept or spin out further, or not; the entire culture and especially pop music—because of its accessibility—were a boundless source of references for me. By chance, David Bowie had guessed my name in "Space Oddity" (1969) and then, pleased at the fortuitous find and also foreshadowing my junkie future, he'd repeated it in "Ashes to Ashes" in 1980, which a little later inspired Peter Schilling's NDW hit "Major Tom (Coming Home)" (1983). The song "Sex Crime (Nineteen Eighty-Four)" (1984) by Eurythmics shed light in euphoric beats on the violence in my childhood home and on the surveillance apparatus around me, while Madonna was so totally in love with me she included my name secretly so it could only be heard at high volume, with her panting it into every horny verse and using the riveting sexualization to establish and develop her position as a pop star. The Smashing Pumpkins, on the other hand, asked me to reach back just a little, to before "1979," where we would meet up.

It was in every song, on every track, even in the dark electro-romanticism of Fever Ray, whose siren songs in "Coconut" addressed me by name and invited me in German to continue doing what I was doing, "jerk them all off" (of course disguised as a just barely perceptible proposal of marriage). The songs by ... "And You Will Know Us" by the Trail of Dead were all greetings from Conrad in Austin (*Will you write again for me?*), and Conrad wasn't just asking if I would write again for him, especially for him, he was asking about when exactly the feelings had stopped and the writing begun, who had bade me stop this living art and whether I'd now completely forgotten myself and no longer even fucking knew who I was. The grief epics by Nine Inch Nails on the other hand identified with me in a painful way (*You can't help my isolation*), with torment in its purest paranoid form poured into sugary dark melodies. Or once walking through Cologne with the otherwise not-much-appreciated Kings of Leon in my headphones, the line *This could be the end* thrumming in the channels of my ears and the windings of my brain made me long for a quick end to this trip: please let's just get there. It was ghostly that Jochen Distelmeyer addressed me directly in the lyrical images he used in the prologue "Eines Tages" (Once upon a Day) to the album *Old Nobody*, rather difficult as a German: "One day / You'll forget him / Step out of the shadows and see you're alone / They weren't ghosts."

The way pop songs address *you*, the *you* forms that turn the listener into an empty space, a variable, was perfectly calibrated to add mini-jolts to my paranoia. Every *you* could be *me*, and so I was constantly being courted, attacked, despised, or loved—whichever way I turned, whatever I listened to. The shuffle function became my oracle, and it seemed that more and more hidden scraps of German could be discerned in the special effect–prone pop English, scraps of the forbidden language from the "land of a thousand guilts." Eminem, "The Way I Am." Chilly Gonzales, "Take me to Broadway." David Bowie, "Hallo Spaceboy." PJ Harvey, "Rid of Me." Archive, "Fuck U." Kate Bush,

"Wuthering Heights." Madonna, "Celebration." Massive Attack, "Inertia Creeps." Leslie Feist, "Mushaboom." The xx, "VCR." Bushido, "Sonnenbank Flavour." Yeah Yeah Yeahs, "Zero." Rihanna, "Umbrella." Tocotronic, "17." Tocotronic, "This Boy Is Tocotronic." Thom Yorke, "Harrowdown Hill." Camille, "Pâle Septembre." Prince, "I Would Die 4 U." Michael Jackson, "They Don't Care About Us." Michael Jackson, "Stranger in Moscow."

The Beatles, the Stones, the Doors.

Justice.

Everyone's entire opus from all time.

Everything, everything, everything.

14

A more detailed example: "Ich Hab's Gesehen" (I Saw It) by Kante. I heard in this a lyrical reminiscence about a weekend in 2001 that Knut and I spent in Hamburg visiting Aljoscha, who was doing a TV internship; it was just before September 11 and right in the middle of the mayoral election campaign. I figured Peter Thiessen, the singer and songwriter, had been watching us and years later decided to contribute to the great counter-enlightenment by writing this song.

"It was a thrill / It was a party / I saw the carnival parade through the streets of Hamburg": the three of us, all guys from the Rhineland and therefore probably ruffian carnivalists from a snooty Hanseatic perspective, had laid down a spectacular, completely blissed-out weekend; we'd stopped in all the bars and clubs that counted, including Pudel and Tanzhalle St. Pauli, and when it turned out to be too early for the fish market in the morning we headed for the big market hall where we could think of nothing better to do than buy an entire box of bananas. We rode to the central train station with this box and started handing out bananas to the morning commuters; they were hesitant at first but seized the opportunity once we added the hastily concocted slogan "Bananas against Schill," an unpopular right-wing politician at the time, literally yanking the fruit out of our hands, one banana after the other. It was a real carnival, and oddly enough the station tramps, who were just as drunk as we were, were the ones who mouthed off noisily in protest. The commuters grinned and benefited.

"I saw the uninvited guests / At the golden buffets": our reputation as hotel crashers probably preceded us, the same way everything had preceded me my entire life, whoever I was and whatever I did. We'd often snuck breakfasts at the buffets of the grand hotels in Berlin, swindling our way in posing as rock stars and using room numbers we'd checked out beforehand, to then chow down on mackerel and macchiatos after dancing the night through. Once Knut laughed so hard he fell off his chair. We'd fought hard for all that, and Thiessen knew how to sing a song about it.

"I saw the devil doubt himself / And the sour milk in the tea": obviously referring to me. The devil, on the go for as long as humankind can remember, forever a counterweight to God, a fantasy figure, a seducer and the administrator of the evil that often ends up setting goodness free: the creative power of destruction. But also a poor devil, collapsing at the edge of the dance floor when intoxication tips into depression, cowering melancholically at the edge of the train station, with the anti-Schill banana in hand, staring out into the void, turning over eternal self-doubts. The "sour milk in the tea" was a contrasting, milder image: a shot of indigestion with regard to high culture, my life already spooled off and turning sour, maybe poisonous— or was Thiessen actually sitting there when I told Knut and Aljoscha about the lumpy milk in my aunt's teacup?

"I saw it / I was there": countering all indirect reports, versions, rumours, and mis-tellings—the insistence on eye witnesses. He saw us, he really can report, and he presents his knowledge in rather blurry but suggestive images.

"And if I want / I will go back / I know the tricks / The secret word / I know the way / 'Cause I was there": a subliminal message for me, a nod after the glance into the abyss. Also a confession that it's possible for the madness we spread around to take hold of us again, if we want it to. The "key word" acquires a central function: it's not just a code word that provides access to some dark party, it emphasizes complicity in writing that will once again conjure up the absolute moment, make things dance and burst, like in Novalis's "Then will our whole inverted being / Before a secret word be fleeing."

I interpreted everything within seconds and according to my obsessions. Other songs, mostly by Trail of Dead but also ABBA, U2, and other groups were far more concrete, named actual years and possible meeting points. I could fill a whole book with such misinterpretations. Shreds of them keep resonating when I hear the songs in the street or in some bar, and I briefly remember how things used to be when the whole world consisted only of feedback. I can trigger this paranoia and once more understand how awful it was. Because if I want to, I can go back. I know the tricks, the secret word. I know the way. *'Cause I was there.*

15

Then came the premiere in Jena. I prowled around the theatre before the performance, went into the theatre café, tried to lift a bottle of whisky, and got caught. They treated it as a joke. I had a beer, I waited, the performance started, and I went backstage. Marvin calmed me down and at every bit of laughter from the audience I put an imaginary mark on the wall. I recently heard, years later, that even during the show and with the actors in full costume, I'd kept hammering them with criticism; I was following a blur of the performance on a monitor. The actors really hated me. When it was time to take the bow at the end, I remember yanking everyone a step forward with the words, "That was me," to remind the group holding hands of what they had just acted in: the consciousness of the world. There lay vanity, so open, so bare, and so sick.

16

Now I was one of those I had earlier considered the undead. Someone in exile, no longer alive, who belonged in the alpine resort I'd imagined years earlier for Thomas Bernhard, Samuel Beckett, and Sarah Kane. Where would I find it? I could hardly feel myself anymore, I'd been silenced and set aside in a parallel world. No reactions reached me anymore.

I wanted to take account of this, describe it. Some of the undead had probably had similar experiences: they'd had to take refuge in a faked death because in life they were cast out into a nether world. It became clear to me that not every case had been voluntary.

I posted my obituary on my blog ("our dear companion in the struggle has passed on") and manipulated my Wikipedia entry, which I had never touched before, to say I'd been shot dead in Leipzig by a policeman. For a few hours I was officially dead.

A telephone avalanche. Hauke was the first to get the news and phoned Robert and Aljoscha right away. They thought it was serious and notified the police. The police broke into my apartment and found nothing, since I was in Leipzig, my cell phone switched off. The rumour of my death also came up in some forum, where people admitted outright that they weren't actually happy to hear about it, but still…Yeah, but what? But yes, maybe they were.

I was hanging out at the train station in Leipzig, Eminem in my ears, stretched out on a bench watching people's spindly legs stalk by. I actually felt I was in the beyond, living in a completely different space from the rest of humanity, stuck in some gap in the wall. I was dead, no longer perceptible, a spirit. So that's what it felt like.

When I got back to Berlin my apartment door was open. The circular hole where the lock used to be looked brutal. I couldn't tell: had state security been there? Anything was possible; nothing was important.

Except: I had now provided them with a legal solution. They could interpret my obituary as a threat to commit suicide, even though I had no such intention, located in the nether world as I was. But now that the risk of self-harm was official, it was possible to commit me against my will, force me into a psych ward, and keep me there as long as they wanted. Which is what happened.

17

I met Aljoscha in a bar called Trödler (Junk Store), and Hauke soon joined us. They checked me out, probably had a short talk outside, which I hardly registered, then kept me in place with beer and questions. I let rip, told them whatever. Nothing was reaching me anymore.

Then the actual kidnapping took place. Suddenly there were policemen in the bar. Aljoscha himself was surprised at how many there were. "So many?" he exclaimed. An entire squadron in full riot gear if I remember correctly, real emergency fighters in heavy protective clothing. Or were there just five or six street cops? They'd probably mis-understood the word *bipolar*.

Even then, at a moment when I was truly out of it, I found the incident embarrassing. The barman and the other customers looked at me in dismay. I was led out. Outside, Aljoscha said again how shocked he was that there were "so many pigs," a choice of words the cops didn't appreciate. They'd come in response to his call, so could he cut out the name-calling, okay?

The police were actually a little helpless. Maybe the word *bipolar* had made them imagine a new variant of Islamism. If I remember correctly, I got in the car without them put-ting handcuffs on me. Next to me, in the driver's seat, was a pretty blond policewoman wearing a name tag that let me use her name for the jokes that, strangely enough, I kept making, one after the other. *Frau Hauenhorst* ("Ms Bushbeater"), *you just did a great job of beating that light, we'll have to drink to that later; Frau Hauenhorst, you turn right up ahead, I know the way.* She kept having to chuckle, friendly and open. The streetfighters sitting in the back were grumpily silent. They probably wondered what kind of an idiot they'd arrested. Or saved?

18

At the Urban Hospital they gave me a dose of medication that put me completely out of commission for the next few days. I don't know anything more about it, and I didn't know then, either. They used a big hit of Haldol, and who knows what other antipsychotics and sedatives, to knock me out. It was awe-inspiring.

"Pretty brutal, the way they sedated you," Dr Neumann, the doctor in charge, said a few weeks later when he read the report. By that time, I'd already forgotten. Time was gone, and I spent many days just drifting around in a semi-twilight. The quasi-realm I'd constructed in my mind, the gap I was inhabiting between life and death had now reached my brain in plain neurochemical ways. Its hyperactivity had been killed right off. I was probably slobbering.

But resistance returned. I painted the entire surface of one of the tables in the smoking room, sketched out a huge map of the world that I marked up with the locations of certain pop bands. Johanna, who paid me a visit that day, described it two years later: I'd settled the Beatles over in New York and Tocotronic were waiting somewhere near the North Pole. One of the nurses got very angry at my "graffiti." So I made a futile attempt to erase the enormous picture. I took photos of the barred windows and used them as nice frames for my blog, where my writing, and therefore my life, were trapped. I could access the blog with my smartphone, which they'd forgotten to take away. Of course, the blog was no longer a blog, only a mad flickering, with sometimes meaningless messages I would delete and replace with a song or strange photos. At some point I deleted it completely. And at four o'clock every morning I'd be sitting in the smoking room, smoking, thinking, reading this and that. The cleaning lady who started work at five and always exchanged a few words with me, called me "Dream Man" when she mentioned me to one of the nurses, the one I figured was the sister of the journalist Peter Richter just because of her last name. That made us laugh. I liked the cleaning lady, and I suppose she liked me.

19

Oddly enough this stay in a psych ward was one of the most profitable in my now rather impressive career in psychiatry. Though *profitable* is hardly the right word. Still, in spite of the usual horror of a closed ward, and in spite of the chemically instigated helplessness I was reduced to, I have kept a few positive memories of this time. And that is due to two or three other patients.

There was Czaikowski, a man of about sixty-five, who I couldn't really read at first. He smoked cheap cigarillos and stoically stared out the window, sticking his nose up in the air and wrinkling it like a proud dog who sees something in the distance that no one else can see. He exuded a tranquillity quite uncommon for such a place. You could hardly see any signs of illness in him. And when he got into a conversation, he would usually end it with an aphorism. When he told me why he was there—his ex-wife had stolen all his savings so he'd wanted to hang himself, "I didn't want to keep going"— he added, with a downward gesture, "Down there, in the ground, it's cold." Then he gave me a glance that went from meaningful to amused, turned his gaze back to the window and into the distance, took a drag on his cigarillo, and wrinkled his nose. That's what his aphorisms were like. I didn't quite understand: was it a good thing that the temperature of a grave was rather wintry? Didn't matter. It was probably some kind of prospect. Maybe cold meant peace. Maybe not. The mere fact that he spoke in aphorisms provided comfort.

Czaikowski had already had a full life that included his escape from East Germany across the Spree River, a story he recounted in detail. He'd strapped his first wife, now deceased, on his back, and had almost drowned in the process. But they'd made it. I was foggily amazed. Then he fell silent and looked at me, amused, until his gaze again drifted casually to the sky outside. Czaikowski was the island of calm, who simply through his presence, his attentiveness, could impose peace, which is why a certain harmony set in whenever he entered the room and absorbed the mood. I was always happy to see him. And thanks to Lina we got to know each other a little.

Because Lina talked to everybody, hooked us all up, until she alienated everybody again. She was a whirlwind, constantly on the move, explosive, almost epileptic, her steps yearning to square the circle. She was a special case, and so had a room of her own which she was often not allowed to leave. Then we'd talk on the doorstep. Or she'd squat there on the doorsill as though she were in starting blocks at a racetrack, a rakish grin on her face, her arms streaked with cutting scars. I called her "tiger girl" which made her crack up. She was in her mid-twenties, had an angular Otto Dix face and wolf's teeth and was always high energy, a junkie from Kottbusser Tor. She was intelligent, far too quick for the others, far too impulsive. They put restraints on her, and we could do nothing about it. When she ranted about the caregivers, who supposedly accused her of having sexual relations with half of the patients, you couldn't tell what was true. In fact, she was in a relationship with one of the patients, if you can call it that, and as a joke she'd also use his name for me, and crow about how she'd rarely had as many boyfriends as she did here. There were "Frankies" everywhere! Her basic goodness was under constant attack from her hysteria. Borderline, they said. Heroin addiction, they said. When I asked Dr Neumann about her, he sighed and said, yes, life often took it out on the talented ones. It was the same in my case, I had this illness and the illness sometimes tripped me up, and that was shitty. That's exactly how he said it: the best, the simplest line I ever heard from the mouth of a doctor in my entire hospital career.

Lina was great for spinning fantasies. Once we were sitting on one of the tables in the dining room, gazing out of the second-storey window onto the snow-covered meadows that sloped down to the frozen Landwehr Canal and were strewn with small black figures. "Ooh, this is great, we're on our sleds," she said, and I actually felt that sudden jerk, the moment when, for a few breaths, the fantasy of sledding became real in a mad attack of acutely free thought. We didn't have to be out there, we could slide down the hills right here, zip down the slopes, play around, and it didn't even feel at all as though it was happening only in our heads. The hill was right out there in front of us. The hill was at our feet.

Gökhan was one of the friendliest people I have ever met but you couldn't talk to him, he was so locked up in his own world. And his world revolved around only one question: *How many children do I actually have?* He didn't know, he couldn't know. He was maybe nineteen years old, corpulent, a younger, baby elephant version of Danny DeVito, and he sat there, smiling happily whenever you talked to him. Then he'd start right in, babbling into himself and sometimes at you, totally happy at how little he knew about his breeding biography: "Dunno how many kids I got. Six hunderd? Seven hunderd 'n' ten? Dunno!" And I understood. A guy really couldn't know. How could you ever know what might happen in a one-night stand? I started doing the math myself. How often had I had sex? And how many children might I have? I had no idea!

When you're crazy you often recognize other people's craziness, but your own remains quite invisible. I told one girl who thought Osama bin Laden was her father that it was absolutely not true, but at the same time I suspected I was the son of the pop star Sting. Quite the party, and I had a pretty good time with these uprooted crazies. Of course, the usual inventory of a psychiatric ward was there too, people who were not only crazy but malevolent, or totally got on your nerves (and how often had I been part of that group!), even though a small kernel of goodness might still flare up in them. The hideous little pimp, for instance, who would pace up and down the corridor with his idiotic silent cow of a girl-friend on his arm and his Andy Capp hat on sideways, strolling along as though they were on some boulevard and yelling out random prohibitions and rebukes against the other patients. I encountered him once later, by chance in Dahlem, where he was required to report to some social agency and he suggested we should meet up sometime, he could supply coke and women, only the best. I just shook my head and said, "Let's." And then there was the flabby round giant who I thought was either a Nazi or a child molester, who didn't say a word, just grinned awkwardly at nothing and ate like a pig. The ethereal young guy who claimed that Sven Marquardt, the famous bouncer at Berghain, had helped him out so much, helped him out so much, and repeated this to people three times a day, including to Lars von Trier, who I thought was also one of the patients. I was pissed off that von Trier kept clinging to me so I refused to say a single word to him.

At some point Czaikowski was moved out to an institution in the suburbs, into assisted housing. That was fine with him and he wrinkled his nose and winked at us as he said goodbye. Lina, on the other hand, was being restrained more and more often. Once there were ten caregivers and security people around her, forcing her to the ground. I couldn't do anything about it. The scene was extremely brutal and sent the whole ward into shock.

I hope they're still alive. I like thinking about them.

20

Once there was a quarantine. Some infectious disease was circulating. One by one, we were confined to our rooms, which became singles during this period, for a day or two. Anyone who came in had to wear a mask, lab coat, and gloves. Of course I saw it all as a sham, and this was supported by Ingo Niermann who happened to come for a visit while I was in quarantine. I consider Niermann a clever prankster who produces brilliant effects on his travels through the deserts, tropics, and dictatorships of this world, effects that are both fake and hyperreal. Now he was sitting there across from me wearing a mask and a lab coat as though in some contaminated developing country or bad sci-fi movie. Very fake, very hyperreal. What a masquerade in the name of truth.

I didn't believe anything, doubted everything, daily came to a dozen wrong conclusions that led nowhere. But I said nothing, and slowly recovered my strength. Little by little I managed to convince the doctors that my death notice had been a joke and not a threat to commit suicide. There was no risk of me harming myself, I explained to them. Which was true. In order to present them with completely waterproof argumentation I'd procured a copy of the relevant legislation and learned it almost by heart. I'd also bought copies of the German Civil Code and the Criminal Code, which I studied erratically. My latest idea was that I was actually a lawyer, and that one day I would see to it that all the violations the state had perpetrated against me and many others were accounted for and made good. My mania, though somewhat dimmer, was still having its effects. And so they loosened the fetters. They let me go to my apartment quite often, which I wanted to develop into a sealed-off artist's cell. No one would be allowed in, I thought. I lay on the mattress and hankered after freedom. My thoughts were confused, but one thing was clear: I didn't want to go back. Lina had been sedated out of reach and restrained to total silence, Czaikowski housed elsewhere. Why go back? I'd noticed that they didn't follow up on the occasional patient who stayed away. They just let it go. And why not? They didn't always have to get the police involved. This wasn't a forensic unit. So why shouldn't I just stay away?

21

I don't remember how I did it, whether I just didn't return one day or discharged myself against the advice of the doctors. In the end, the result was the same. At some point I was back in my apartment, nervous, highly nervous, in no way coherent, quite the contrary. The excess medication had only managed to temporarily stuff the attack back into the holes it had emerged from and temporarily plaster them over. Now it came bursting through again, under pressure, and the illness that had been anaesthetized for awhile exploded into full bloom. I posted insane things on the web and powered through the days and the streets like an uncertain detonation, more and more enraged at nothing in particular. And there was a new deadline bearing down on me. I had just forgotten about it.

In February I'd given notice on my apartment. I'd come to realize that this so-called studio, a trashed dive, was no longer worthy of me and I'd never been happy there anyway. So I'd given notice, just like that, wham. Then I forgot about it, or when I did think about it, quickly set it aside— something else would come up, and besides I had so much to do every day. I would end up being very rich anyway and would just *buy* something.

This unfortunate step, among all the other unfortunate steps, had particularly serious consequences, and soon led to a weird form of exile. Basically, this exile has continued to this day.

Then they arrested me.

22

This is not an arrest, Karl-Uwe yells at me and the policemen as he comes down the staircase in his dressing gown. Oh yeah, what is it then? "This is not an arrest," he yells again, at our backs as they lead me away. I figure that's supposed to calm me down. Petra from across the landing comes running through the courtyard, kisses me on the cheek, and assures me that she loves me. That, too, is meant to give me strength. As we step out onto the street and two passersby observe the scene, I feel like Johnny Cash in the iconic 1965 photograph. The eyes of the passersby are the camera. Cash was arrested in El Paso for drug smuggling and the photo looks staged, too cool, too handsome to not have been set up, with handcuffs that look like some especially casual accessory. And they're all wearing sunglasses, the marshals and Cash too. We're not wearing sunglasses. We're not cool either. And the handcuffs, I realize now, are just a disgrace. I am not Cash, I am myself, and this is just another disaster.

They push me into the police car, the cop's hand presses me down so that I won't hit my head, but it is also an expression of power, you get the picture. One of the policemen says he has to detain the handcuffs again. "Detain" is what he actually says but the word isn't right. "Detain" implies bringing someone into the station and checking their ID. But yes, he insists, he'll have to "detain" the handcuffs. Maybe I used the word myself, mistakenly, and he is now taking it up as a joke. The handcuffs are already so tight I ask why he has to make them even tighter; he says *detain.* He fiddles around with the screws, fastens the handcuffs down till they cut into my flesh. Then we drive off. Up front they're talking a Slavic language I can't understand. I let it all happen. There's probably some reason. They take me to the Urban Hospital.

What happened? Music. I'd been listening to music. It was loud. My old system had burned out long ago and so I'd run the music via the TV and a DVD player. What else? I don't know. They knocked, it was before ten at night, actually it was half past nine, which I can check in the relevant issue of *Dummy*. I opened the door. They looked at me for two, three seconds. I looked back. Then, without a word, they grabbed hold of my hands, pushed me up against the wall, and snapped on these handcuffs that will probably accompany me for the rest of my life.

I ask, "What's the problem? Is there a complaint against me?"

The policeman responds, "Thousands of complaints."

The dark city moves past outside, the facades, the traffic lights, the dark glaze all over the concrete. It's shimmering and sparking and roaring. Soon I'll be back in jail.

23

Something else happened, earlier. One morning I woke up in a particularly trembly condition. A fit of rage hurled me out of bed. I stood there not knowing what would come next. I snatched the stack of letters from the desk and leafed through them. A letter from an office caught my attention. It mentioned a summons to appear before a judge, a woman, somewhere near Möckernbrücke. They were going to revoke something? My citizen's rights? They were going to sic caregivers on me. I went downstairs and threw the letter in the recycling (screwed-up people sort garbage too). Then I fished it out again and set it on fire. I am not sure why but a strange impulse made me tuck the burning paper back in the garbage container. Would it burn? Was this still real? I tacitly accepted that the container would burn up but at the same time I wanted to put out the fire. I scooped the burning papers out of the container but the embers had spread. I spit in the container. Didn't work. It was on fire. I wanted to go get some water upstairs but that would take too long, the garbage would be up in flames. A guy I'd never seen before came up and tried to help put out the fire. He had a bottle of water with him. "You trying to burn us all up, man?" he muttered. I shook my head, no, not at all. The fire kept burning and melted a hole into the bottom of the blue plastic bin, creating little bubbles. Somehow the guy and I did it. The fire was out, but there were still embers. A column of smoke over Kreuzberg. I thought about how they announce the election of a new pope, *habemus papam*, and went up to my apartment. I had a guilty conscience, felt like confessing, but I hadn't believed in that sacrament for a long time, and don't believe in it now as I write either.

24

Something else had happened earlier. A tenant, a woman in the apartment below me, moved out. The day she was moving I came across her on the stairs, on my way home from one of my city excursions, and offered to help her friends carry boxes.

She flipped out. "It's not for you to help me move!"

"Why not?"

"I'm moving out because of you, man!"

That was news to me. I didn't understand.

One of her friends saw the expression on my face and said, "Now I'm on his side."

I didn't even know there were sides. We'd had nothing to do with each other. She'd never complained about the loud music.

I must have creeped her out so badly.

25

And something else had happened earlier, and something else too. Something happened every day in fact. But these events merged into one another, turning into a single blurry film still. I'm in the police car, we'll be there soon. Yes, they're taking me to the Urban and not to jail. I tell myself I'm relieved. Then the reception in emergency, one of many such receptions, I can hardly tell them apart anymore. Upstairs they medicate me again, intravenously. And I'm gone.

I'm gone for the next weeks.

No memory.

26

No, there's one doctor, a woman from the SPD, the social-psychiatric service, I vaguely remember. "There's a fire, Herr Melle, a fire!" is what she'd shout at me in the corridor of the closed ward. Sometimes she had her teeth in, sometimes she didn't.

"You've been hanging around in front of women's apartments!" she yelled. I'd completely forgotten about that. I'd been invited to a reading by a group of theatre people, among them a woman director I vaguely knew. Something had set me off, maybe the snotty way the invitation was formulated. I'd gone to the group's studio and knocked on the door in a rage, and when no one opened up I'd left a letter that was probably confused and nasty. Even though I actually liked these people.

When the toothless doctor appeared on her weekly rounds in the ward only to read her patients the riot act, she reminded me of this incident, and for a brief moment I realized that there was something wrong with me, and quite massively. It made me hesitate and feel guilty. Being locked up in a closed ward didn't have that effect at all. I ascribed that to the secret hostility toward the state they all said I displayed, a hostility the state returned in kind. But now that people I knew and had worked with in the theatre were apparently notifying authorities that I was a danger, I got thinking.

Then a new blast of neuron fire burned away those doubts.

27

I have already described how, in my case, manic outbreaks come with a sort of Jesus-fantasy, a saviour complex that can take pretty bizarre forms, making me think I have to share the burdens of all the sick and forgotten people in the world; they are, after all, sick and forgotten because of me. I have to offer refuge to all those who are lost, distressed, faltering, those who are suffering and alienated from life, even if it is only a virtual refuge, an imaginary one, constructed in fictions, in just one word I might utter. It can be a phrase I notice in a book, or a song, or a post or blog; I ponder it and in my thoughts I offer help, sometimes even make contact. But language has become unreliable, coded into grotesque forms, thoughts are twisted, and so such notices from me arrive elsewhere as threats rather than offers of help, especially where women are concerned. The fact that a manic person feels irresistible and that subconsciously there may also be amorous motivations gives the whole thing a disastrous twist. From there it is not far to the stalker, and such accusations are still whirring around in the world and on the web today. In my experience, it does no good to explain that you were ill or to apologize. Some people seem to want to cling to these stories and forget that despite all his manic missteps there is a human being at the other end who has been fighting a bloody battle, a battle against his own blighted blood.

28

The weeks were shot to pieces by antipsychotics. I don't remember how I got out. Rather than see the psychiatric ward as a place to get better, the patient sees it as a jail they need to break out of. Now I was completely without ties, social contacts had dissolved, probably because I wanted it that way, I pushed people away. I had no contact with Aljoscha anymore. There were other visitors but fewer and fewer, understandable since those visits can be extremely unpleasant for the visitor. You don't bring a friend who broke his leg a bouquet of flowers. You're an unwelcome misery-tourist in the centre of all the creepiness and you get nothing but abuse from the creeps there. Some people can't handle that, and I understand. Maybe I couldn't either.

I zoomed around town as a truly free radical and became more and more unpredictable. I travelled to Cologne to some literature event even though I usually avoid such affairs. I was supposed to do a reading. This reading, too, turned into a partial fiasco. I arrived late because I'd missed the train again, I smoked even though it was forbidden, I provided rude and meaningless answers, almost wrecked the microphone. If Patrick Hutsch, the moderator, hadn't been so level-headed I would probably have acted out even more. I thought it was absurd that my mother, my aunt, and her husband showed up for the reading. And I mouthed off to the organizers for no reason. In the evening I (actually) shook hands with Patti Smith, said hello to the feminist Alice Schwarzer, and in the morning I told Roger Willemsen something stupid about Charlotte Roche, sat down at the piano in the foyer of the hotel, and played like hell. I hardly need mention that I can't play piano.

I stayed in Cologne an extra two days, living in the Chelsea Hotel because I was infected with Martin Kippenberger again, and I knew he'd made one of his deals with the hotel owner: art in return for a room. What Kippenberger could do, I could do even better, and so after two days of straying around I left my journal full of scribbles in the room and took off without paying.

29

It was noon and I was out in front of the Berghain nightclub. Years earlier, Aljoscha and I had been there often, before the hype, amazed at the deep thrum in this sublime cathedral of steel. Now I was back in front of the place, with author Helene Hegemann's *Axolotl Roadkill* in my hand, oddly enough, a book I felt was a gift but that also struck me as poisonously infested with the parlance of the Volksbühne Theatre. I could hardly stand reading it. It was embedded in the pervasive Pollesch lingo that had long infiltrated the conversations of my friends and worked well for people who wanted to come across as know-it-alls and deny their identities. Really, though, it was just a pimped-up way to express hollow consent for the socially validated smart-speak of the moment. In the hall of mirrors that was subversively veiled bourgeois life, people assured each other they were experiencing harmless alienation but then carried right on, merrily consolidating it all. And even kept winking at each other.

I stood there, no lineup anywhere. Sven Marquardt came out, looked me over, and glancing at the book wanted to know if I'd come to celebrate Hegemann's birthday, or what? That made me laugh. He grinned and waved me in.

Inside, a deep dark rampaging paradise awaited me. The music pressed into every pore. I became a function of the music. Mad impulses came from somewhere and drove right through me. Somewhere something seemed to be *calculating* and *pumping*. It was driving and funnelling me straight down into this organism of steel and flesh, following the bass along channels into every corner and right to the middle of the dance floor, whamming its joy straight in my face. I downed two or three drinks, my brain shaken up by the music, I danced in time with the beat. I joined some girls I didn't know, zapping back and forth, high-five, high-five. Had some long drinks and some beer, lost myself in the beat, loved the music, felt like euphorically smashing open my head against the walls that were pearling with sweat. Lost fifty euros in the cigarette machine, didn't matter, kept on dancing, kissed somebody. Danced some more, sat somewhere, talked, stood up, walked, then danced, finally got comfortable on a kind of pyramid, almost a throne. Round about me, the women found room to spread out like mermaids at my feet, they lay down on the altar of Neptune. I was agleam because I wanted to be. Associations with Greek mythology set in, gorgeous demigods, fates, and nymphs, water games where there was no water, an air-aquarium. Wordless, the animals came together, coupled, and went their ways, painlessly. Something ur-archaic was at work here, and I was melding in with it.

I must have spent twenty-four hours in there.

Then I spotted Picasso and flew into a rage. It's hard to imagine how crazy someone must be if they can fantasize about catching sight of a major, long-deceased artist of the previous century in a Berlin techno club. So Picasso was sitting on the toilet, talking thick-tongued, with some metrohipsters; he was wearing a belt whose buckle spelled out F.U.C.K. in gold letters. He had a particularly virile-gay look about him, and when I stopped in front of him he gazed at me with his round, childlike, searching eyes. I immediately got mad. What was he doing here? With no further thought

I dumped my red wine in his lap. That would cool down the artist of the century!

Why red wine at all? I ask myself today, I hardly ever drink wine. Maybe the ancient Greek vibe of the club had seduced me into imbibing the grape. Picasso lost it, of course, and came bounding after me. I took off. He chased me up the stairs, and down the stairs, and I finally thought, dammit, if you're going to do stupid stuff, pour fucking wine in Picasso's fucking lap, then you need to face up to it. So I stopped somewhere on a metal platform and coldly stared him in the eye. He made for me, like in a film. We tangled. I'd never liked Picasso, it had all come flowing out of him too organically, too naturally, without pause, without reflection, too banal, a primordial gorging on highly potent honey. Secretly and probably unconsciously I resented what I dubbed his *creanaturalness*. In the end it was nothing but sperm. A security guy separated us and I apologized to Picasso and told the security guard he didn't need to say a thing, I'd had enough now and was leaving the joint voluntarily. And so everyone relaxed. I got my jacket and left.

Picasso. You have to picture that.

30

The megalomaniac boulevard of superstars that I always end up tearing along when I have one of these episodes reveals an obsession with celebrities and personalities that is already out of control when I'm healthy. It speaks of a strange vanity, a yearning for belonging and greatness.

When I was young, there were no role models in my immediate surroundings; everything was boxed-in, small, dreadful, so the role models and stars had to be brought in from afar. I visited the Protestant church library every week, and the volunteer ladies there already intimated *something'll come of him*; whatever was faraway in the books held a promise, a wager for the future, a space that was open to me, a way out of the narrow everyday. After all, artists had turned their weaknesses and limitations into something else, something that opens up, that points beyond them, art, drastic art that took my breath away. I read like crazy and cut myself off more and more. Internal exile, a double life, it may sound like an exaggeration, but early on I understood what that might mean.

Was my youthful fascination with music, literature, and stars already a sign of my later illness? Did these obsessions, and the escapism, already have manic aspects? And the other side of the story, the fact that there is little that touches me or even reaches me today, is that more than just a factor of aging? Is it a result of all the medication that suffocates excessive emotions from the get-go?

Once you're sick, everything becomes suspect.

31

One interesting hypothesis I came across and that immediately made sense connects the outbreak of bipolar disorder with a person's tendency to be overly conformist. In healthy times, the strong internal impulses that such a disposition triggers are strictly suppressed in order for a person to function socially. In fact, the sick person tries to be too forthcoming toward others, doesn't set up appropriate boundaries, feels irritations where no one else does, seeks perfection in fulfilling tasks and duties until, as one expert, Professor Thomas Bock, puts it, they are one day "overpowered" by "all the demands, both external and internal." Then the game is up, and the once so adamant self-discipline breaks into a thousand shards of self-loss.

The feeling that *you're finally really living your life, finally recognizing and raising your own voice* is part of the mania. I've been quiet so far; now it's my turn to talk. I've been tricked out of everything so far; now I'm taking what I deserve. Doesn't matter how: by stealing, or mouthing off, or throwing a fit, and these episodes get more and more intense each time. Faint character traits that simply added shadings to your personality now proliferate into distortions. The internal corset explodes.

I have always tended toward rebelliousness thanks to an exaggerated sense of justice that would emerge as surly opposition when I was in my right mind. My conformism has always been mixed with a complicated wish to be different. With each bout of illness, this beast becomes a monster, and the justice I demand becomes an excess of the ego.

I get slammed back and forth between these two poles: conformism and rebelliousness. I cannot shake off my background and the consequences of that background. Even as an adolescent, I would try to ensure that any resistance on my part was legitimized by brilliant results at school, because it was on the basis of this brilliance that I could make demands. At some point, in my teenage years and in response to some kind of pressure, I gingerly but visibly cut my legs with a razor blade. Nowadays that would be a clear sign of a borderline condition. At the time, that didn't exist, thank god. And nobody noticed, except the gym teacher, and he didn't say anything.

32

Kubrick again. I'm in my apartment, which I will soon have to vacate, and am building a moonscape. This is necessary because something went wrong: yesterday, or the day before that, or maybe last week, I sprayed the logo of my alter ego, "Jean-Christophe von Toulouse Jerkycock," on the wall of the corridor leading to the bath—in bright, garish colours, quite the success. The logo is a hysterical rooster. It consists of a circle with a dot in it, two running legs attached below, two streaks that separate and mark an open, shrieking beak on the left, the coxcomb up top, which is sometimes just a comma, sometimes an expansive, punky rainbow of colours. That's the logo of Toulouse Jerkycock, an Icelandic physicist, smitten by poetry, who is visiting Berlin and blogging Dadaist stuff in a fantasy language.

I am not sure if the name of my alter ego has anything to do with the director Jan-Christoph Gockel ("Christopher Cock"), who is an acquaintance. I don't think so, although such suspicions have been brought forward. I wish to politely reject them here. I may be mistaken but I think I picked up the word *Jerkycock* in a bar called Fuchsbau, when I heard the guy I think is Peter Handke's nephew and who writes the daily lunch specials on the blackboard in perfect script, apply the term to someone else, but in a friendly way. But yes, okay, maybe it does have something to do with Jan-Christoph, but not in regard to content. Because Jan-Christoph is great. But Jean-Christophe von Toulouse Jerkycock is fantastic! Unbeatable! And he's the talk of the town. As the actor Robert Stadlober let me know in a secret whisper he disguised as a cell phone conversation under the Kreuzberg sun, when he told me how much fun he and his friends were having with my creation: "Thanks for the Jerkycock," is what he said with a grin, and added, "Jerkycock, that's me!" And in fact, he looks just like I imagine the Icelandic bird.

But then I decided to paint over the beautiful, shrill picture. I got the white paint I'd bought in advance and covered over the plump rooster. In a hysterical move I accidentally knocked over the paint can. Irritated, I stood there looking at the thick paint ooze along, then decided I needed to stop it and, weirdly, stomped my foot into it, and finally walked defiantly through the whole apartment. I spread the white around. And now I'm using it to create a grand installation, with bedsheets, feathers, more paint, a springboard, and moon craters that I punch into the cheap wallboard with my fist. It's all Hollywood anyway. And nobody can tell me that Kubrick, our moon-landing faker, is dead.

The apartment issue is getting more urgent. I really will have to move out soon. Yeah, so what! Under pressure from my agent I've even looked at two apartments that I didn't much like, or the people didn't like me, or nobody liked anything. And I'm sure I distinctly heard the left-wing-radical-looking landlady at the first place whisper, "I hate you" in my ear. So now I've stopped looking for an apartment.

Something will turn up. It always does. I'm not sure what, or when. But I know that it will. *That* I know for sure. The door the police wrecked is now down on the street, decorated with glyphs and little messages. I wonder how much it's worth? Nobody's taken it away.

33

Sometime later, I carried the door back upstairs, laid it down on the floor, and puttied the hole shut; I glued a chair on it, added a flag, and one night, as a statement, tossed it off the Kottbusser Bridge into the Landwehr Canal, which people on the other side immediately applauded. The strange raft drifted slowly down the canal, approximately in the same area where I'd tossed out the letters to the editor that came in response to my *Zeit* article bashing Celan. I watched the raft slip away and calculated its route.

I was living only in simulations, believing every conspir-

acy theory and not a single one. History was the greatest
fiction ever. Historiography was nothing but a struggle for
my attention, a struggle for me, an experiment of the spirit
of the world that was me. The Holocaust had not actually
taken place. I even believed *that* for a few days. Churchill,
Stalin, Hitler, Chamberlain had all been in cahoots, no
they'd *all* agreed to simulate the catastrophe in order to
forestall the danger of the people of the future creating fake
boundaries to contain the battle that would flare up around
them, dealing with it as a fiction before it even occurred.
Because, I thought, it could not be possible that humanity
had produced something as inhumane as the Holocaust. A
reasonable mind simply could not accept that. I'd always
had the facts in my head. In history class the teacher would
utter the line, "It must never happen again," and give me
a meaningfully ambiguous look, and I would meet Anna-
belle's eyes, the most intelligent beauty in the class, and
somehow we would know, without knowing. I had never
understood the facts, or maybe I had, of course I had, but
I'd never really digested them. And now I knew why.

Human migrations were happening. It was biblical. I
was drowning in it all. How many years had gone by since
the Middle Ages? Which Middle Ages exactly? And how
many people were there anyway? Probably way fewer than
they kept telling us. The Middle Ages were only four gener-
ations ago. Or three? Intolerable, all these thoughts, these
lies. On the news channel N-TV Hitler giggled as he spoke
my name. Another beer.

34

The nearer I come to the present the harder it is for me to
recount all this. Karl Ove Knausgård, everybody's pin-and-
pop-up boy these days—I don't believe a word of what he

writes—says it takes ten years until you can write about an experience. Maybe that's why it's so hard for me. But it may also be because this has been the most brutal psychosis so far, with the broadest and most difficult consequences, the longest one, the worst one. Maybe, too, because I'd become a real idiot. How do you write about yourself as an idiot?

But maybe because it took place only a few years ago. Memory has not yet become history. As it is, my memory has suffered some toxicological damage. With the medication and the alcohol, thought retreated into a permanent and no-longer-dissolvable delirium. Occasionally, if it was really necessary, I still managed to play a role, like an actor, to demonstrate to the world around me that I was still functioning.

It was wild on the inside. And there was hardly anyone left on the outside.

35

The technician at Gravis, where I plunk down my paint-smeared computer, and who responds to my comment that I've been doing some painting at home, laughs and asks, "With the computer?" The teller at the Commerzbank to whom I give a little lecture about why and how I'm off to Harvard and who calls out, "Herr Melle is going to America!" as she opens a bank account for me with a soon-to-be-maxed-out line of credit. The judge, who looks at me skeptically as I look at her skeptically. The friends who put me up for one day, and later for another day, and who have tried to be tolerant and thank me for returning the empties even though they must know I'm doing so because I'm short of cash. The taxi driver on the other side of the street whose gesticulation with a pack of Marlboros (a wave that wasn't even in my direction) I interpret as a gesture of solidarity: *I'm with you.* The taxi driver who says, "Never again Soda Club," when I tell him how hostile the tweens were there, how completely confused they were by the news items hanging in the air that they couldn't understand, floating inside a bubble of perfumed flatulence that permeates everything since smoking is no longer permitted. "One of us is lying, one of us is dying." The junior waiter in Schöneberg, an Italian, who whispers "Jewish faggot" at me as he serves up the pizza. The tramp who announces his suicide at the Friedrichstrasse Station just after Obama takes the escalator right in front of me, turns around, and with an intense look in his eyes has nothing to say. My new passion for wearing *wifebeaters*, those ribbed, rapper-style undershirts, Eminem at the corner. Kicking over a sandwich board in front of Kaffee-Café in Berlin-Mitte, which the journalist Claudius Seidl, waiting for a tram, observes and then teasingly remarks that it looks like I've already had a few early beers. Michael Mühlhaus, the former keyboard player for Blumfeld, who listens to me very attentively one evening in front of the Maria Bar and maybe *doesn't* judge. The realization that whenever people talk about me on the sidewalks and in the cafés these days they're using the code name Thomas Müller; when people talk about me they pretend to be talking about the famous soccer player. At the same time, the dull distant drone of the helicopters surveilling me and keeping me in check: the observer becoming the observed. The woman who encounters me lying exhausted against a pillar in the Leipzig train station reading the biography of Ulrike Meinhof, and who asks me, grinning with her bared Latin American teeth, "Is that your only love?" Transcendental meditation. The idea that Jesus is the prototype of all manics. The spot in Adorno where he recognizes the potential seizure of power in the line "absolutely out of the question," a line that accompanies me as a prototype of all evil: this maelstrom of rejection and exclusion that turns whatever is rejected or excluded into the inevitable. The scared expression on the face of an acquaintance after she hears my steps come slapping up the stairs, and timidly asks if I've been drinking before she slams the door in my face. In Motel One, with Agnes, where I am supposed to calm down; she pays for everything. Non-stop movies and film clips, on all channels, and the mission to still save the young people. Reznor, who saves me when I forget my computer in a hostile café; he's greedily breathing in the vibes and rumours that are hanging in the air and reminds me in that deep voice of his, "You forgot your computer," so that I actually go back to the café and find my computer there. And then artistic director Matthias Lilienthal, at a "Recordplayer" evening with Thomas Meinecke, where I knock the glasses off his nose. Jule Böwe at Helene Hegemann's birthday party in Tresor, to whom I noisily announce a new upcoming play, just for her. Patrick, whom I meet again at Balzer's Dosenmusik, in the company of Diedrichsen and who is so alienated he can hardly utter a word. The guy selling döner kebabs who hands me a dürüm-döner and purrs, "Please forgive me, one more time." And finally the ragged specimen who confronts me on Goltzstrasse and smiles despairingly: "They're taking us all for a ride, understand?"

Understood.

36

And the publisher Suhrkamp. In just a few days I ruined my reputation there, too, caused a small scandal and rendered any further collaboration impossible. In January I was invited to a reception to celebrate the publisher moving to

Berlin but couldn't attend because I'd just been committed. I asked my colleague Nussbaumeder to send a message of congratulations to the editor, that was quite resolutely (and manically) "from the psych ward." It was important to add this information. She responded with the remark, "We'll be dealing with that."

What was that supposed to mean? Nothing. Nobody was dealing with anything. How could they! But this little phrase stuck with me and kept on irritating me. How did the publishing house propose to deal with it? Through esoteric calls to my martyred existence? Through incantations from the publisher Siegfried Unseld? Through thought transmission? My particular editor didn't even come to visit. But then, how could she, she'd just lost her job. The next episodes of the so-called Suhrkamp Soaps were being written. A considerable brain drain had weakened the publishing house and a bizarre court case around ownership had ground it down. The publishing house that had once been the backbone of rational discourse and resistance poetry in the dark years of the Federal Republic was falling apart before our very eyes. And my eyes were teary at the sight.

The move to Berlin was a mistake and now they were even opening shop in Berlin-Mitte to celebrate the mistake. Didn't they know that neurotics go completely crazy in big cities? There was evidence that the bigger the city in which you live, the greater your risk of falling completely psychically ill. It was the month of May, and I, a harried dog, a wandering publisher logo, set out with a beer in my hand and my thinking fired up and full of poison to help inaugurate the new location. And my performance was quite obscure, I even berated my friend Nussbaumeder as a jerk, hardly spoke, bounced from here to there until I finally caught sight of the publisher herself, her arm in a cast.

Her arm in a cast!

Of course it was a fake, I saw that immediately. A fake, a gesture of solidarity, a mockery. As *fake* as the person herself, it seemed to me. In the emotional swell this set off I charged straight at her and, as far as I know, bumped into her back. Or did I crash into the cast? The lies and pretenses had to come to an end; I needed to leave a mark, the protest of the virtuous, and seeing as I was supposedly a pretty radical and crass spirit this mark had to be physical to sever the chain of false signifiers. Then I walked out.

The *Frankfurter Allgemeine Zeitung* reported that "The publisher Ulla Unseld-Berkéwicz arrived late, her arm bandaged after a fall in Zehlendorf. Her good mood was briefly disturbed by an aggressive man—perhaps an author who'd been rejected? It was as though Franz Biberkopf had come down from his hut."

So Franz Biberkopf, the murderer in Alfred Döblin's *Berlin Alexanderplatz*.

In any case, it's a bitter memory, the shame, the impulse to push it away, the resistance. I shudder at the thought.

Two years later she accepted my apology.

37

Something similar happened at a reading by Rainald Goetz a few days later, which I disrupted with jeers and catcalls, spiralling down ever deeper into an agitated beer solitude, appearing in good spirits but actually profoundly dark. Goetz, for whom I'd felt a decades-long obsession that I've now more than overcome, didn't really know what to do; how could he? Or he dealt with it by not dealing with it. To top it off, I had him sign a copy of his book at the end of the presentation. A friend later said it wasn't really so bad, I'd just assumed a Bukowski role and done a pretty good job playing it. That is a friendly interpretation of the event, a more relaxed view of things, which is unfortunately not true. The reaction of rock singer Dirk von Lowtzow, who later on that afternoon hissed a determined, "What nerve!" in my face, is probably more appropriate. Journalist Detlef Kuhlbrodt's view is probably the most apt, though it surprised me because I remember the heckling but not the urge to apologize. Detlef wrote, "Or the colleague who spent every break that afternoon hassling people, though I suspect his pushy offensiveness was due to some psychological trauma and too much drinking. He spent the entire afternoon working himself up into completely obnoxious behaviour, for which he kept apologizing, only to get even more offensive. And later on, he enthused about this being the best ever, most fantastic, reading he'd ever attended."

Ever since, I've had a hard time meeting up with certain people.

Thank god I left the publisher and their premises alone after that.

38

An odyssey began. I moved out of the apartment without making the required repairs. Let them use the deposit money to fix the damage. They always tried to hold on to the deposit anyway, right? Now they had a reason. For a month I moved into a shed an acquaintance owned in Berlin-Mitte. Something had in fact turned up. It was midsummer, and unfortunately, I started firing up the stove with my old manuscripts. I was also listening to really loud music again, and in an attack of paranoia I rigged up a security system of cables and weights to block the door. The neighbours notified the owner and when he came by to check, he unceremoniously threw me out. I was briefly able to find room with a couple I was friendly with and to whom I introduced Stephen Fry's documentary *The Secret Life of the Manic Depressive*. Strange: I was obviously aware that I was sick, why else would I have shown them Fry's self-study? But my awareness was fleeting and affected by volatile moods, so that even in moments of clarity there was no real self-recognition. I was aware of my illness, but then again, at the higher level of controlling my actions, I wasn't.

I abandoned that couple and charged on. Through bars and concerts, especially in Kreuzberg. I ran into Aljoscha at a Gustav concert but I was no longer able to connect with him: he was attending a concert, I was waging war in my mind. A short-lived affair provided shelter for a couple of nights, then she dragged me off to a shared-housing office where I soon found another place to stay, for a month. I wasn't allowed to smoke in the apartment, the landlord said. I spread out my stuff, the remains of what I owned, whatever I had left, and tried to come down to earth. Instead, I flew even higher, had another affair in Bonn with a woman who paid for everything, travelled back and forth, kept on losing myself.

And went even crazier on social networks. I'd always rejected Facebook, but now I had not only one account, the one that had saved me in London, but at least three and was suddenly married to myself. I turned into a troll again, berated people, got excited about things and facts I knew nothing about, misunderstood everything and turned vulgar. I secretly continued to believe that my entire life everybody had been betraying me.

I am still dealing with the consequences of those actions today. People who I meet now are warned by their friends: he's crazy, a fanatic, dangerous even, and in one especially obstinate case, he's a stalker. I accept these charges, I apologize, but I also try to explain that I was sick at the time, that I am probably chronically sick, but that a manic attack made me write and do things I would otherwise never write or do—because of twisted, false perceptions, a temporary madness, and not a chronic personality disorder. Otherwise I wouldn't be able to take a step back today and assess the actions that took place then. That is an enormous difference, and I need to insist on clearly establishing that difference. It only works sometimes.

If people continue to issue warnings about me, it makes me wonder if I am a leper, if I have a serious disease. And I have to respond, yes, I am, and yes, I do.

And inside something hurts, dies off, and turns to stone.

39

How can you ever explain to others what you don't understand yourself? How can you ever make plain that yes, you're the one who did these things, but at the same time, it wasn't you? That is the crack, if not the crevice, inside me that I have to live with and that I sometimes try to plaster shut. It is always there and I cannot fill it. My attempt to lead even a somewhat civil bourgeois existence seems to have failed forever. Okay, I accept that, I'll stick that out right to the end, maybe I'll keep on writing, maybe I won't, it's my only escape. But the whispering goes on, even today, years later, the slander, the character assassination. This is not an illness that elicits empathy, and I don't ask for empathy. I don't want to be indulged, and I don't blame everything on the illness. But a certain flexibility in regard to the sick person, a certain openness and circumspection—

I try not to care, try to see the rest of my life as an experiment in defiance.

40

Love is growing that much more difficult. Attempts at intimacy are weighed down with guilt and deviousness, clouded with thousands of rumours. And anger has to be reined in. I cannot allow myself to get angry anymore. Anger is suspect. Others may be permitted an outburst, but I have to stay quiet. How much is due to my difficult, messed-up, and sociophobic character, and how much to the illness? What is deliberate provocation and what is out-of-control tantrum? Will what I say not always be interpreted as the words of someone who once went crazy and may well be forever crazy? And should I even care?

There is no solution. The boundaries between *original*, *inappropriate, strange*, and *sick* are blurry. What applies to others does not apply to me.

I rein in my disdain and make myself up as a freak.

I am finished.

41

Am not.

42

If you only knew what that said before.

43

The landlord came in, I was lying in bed, drunk and wiped out. He had a friend with him and started yelling what was all this *garbage* lying around. And I'd been smoking in the apartment, he could smell it. He could see I was crazy of course, and he gave me an ultimatum of three days to move out.

My friend Anja took over. It was as though the baton from a relay race was hanging in the air somewhere, and every now and then someone would actually grab hold of it. With the decisive energy of the film director she would later become, Anja created temporary order. She confronted the landlord, she got a doctor-friend to assign me a place in the addiction ward of the St. Hedwig Hospital in Berlin-Mitte. She persuaded me to go there and check in. The addiction clinic might not be the most appropriate but the psychiatric team there was good, she said, and what I needed was rest. I was homeless, of course, and this was Anja's way of ensuring I would have a roof over my head. And be in medical care.

She packed up my things with amazing energy and action. Jittery, I could hardly help, and simply admired the speed with which she worked. We rented another moving van, and I stashed my things in a container in the western part of the city.

44

I had become completely destitute. I was supposed to be writing a play for the Wuppertal theatre, but I kept postponing delivery of the text. I'd come up with a sci-fi scenario around Alan Turing, had already titled the play "Touring," and bought numerous books by Philip K. Dick, read bits of them, leafed through them, set them aside. I'd called on the terminally ill media theorist Friedrich Kittler (during the meeting his secretary hissed, "Here's another one of these assholes," into the phone), and discussed a gender-theoretical approach to the Turing test with him. I thought I could write the play in three days. I couldn't. I accomplished little more than a few sketches of Turing himself, got caught up in his biography, and wrote about three pages of Dadaist dialogue. I soon sold all the books and essay collections again, most of which were only vaguely related to the topic, for a fraction of their original cost.

At some point the theatre gave up and the team found another project.

Anja came to visit every day, she brought me the cigarettes my mother was paying for with bank transfers. I continued to hold forth grandiosely, tossing around theories and witticisms as we sat smoking in the spacious courtyard. Actually, she would be sitting, I would be standing and gesticulating, and also berating her. But otherwise I grew quiet in that ward. I hated it there, couldn't find any access to the poly-toxico-maniacs and drunks holed up there. At one point, four of us had to spend a couple of nights together in a room for two. I didn't sleep a wink.

After only two days, one of the caregivers said that my withdrawal symptoms seemed to have disappeared, if they had ever existed. It was true, I was not an addict. But I still spent four weeks in this ward. And my madness had still not abated.

45

"*Clinical report:* Good general condition. Heart: 2/6 systolic murmur, no bruits. Lungs: normal breathing with good bilateral air entry. Abdomen: bowel sound normal, soft to palpation, no organomegaly. Kidneys: no flank pain. No signs of vascular inflammation. Pulses intact."

The actress Malenka also came to visit, which made me happy. I remembered going for a walk with her in Monbijou Park and how conscious I was of *stepping out.* Just weeks earlier I'd been on a short trip to Vienna with Malenka, which had also ended in such a catastrophe I hardly want to recall it. We'd visited the grave of Falco and the Thomas Bernhard Clinic at Steinhof. Literally raced up the airy Baumgartner Heights at a crazy tempo, as I later heard, with her in a melodramatically billowing coat and me talking non-stop. We'd stayed with a couple of drama-turges, friends of Malenka. We'd gone out for Chinese food.

But suddenly, the second night there, it all struck me as so false that I threw a temper tantrum. I yelled and screamed at the entire world. Malenka tried to calm me down but couldn't. I don't remember why I got so angry. It must have had something to do with the sclerotic bour-geois environment I was in, and with the fact that nothing was working the way I wanted. Although in my constantly mutating mind I hardly knew what I wanted or how things were meant to work. Work? What does that mean, work? What exactly?

Malenka couldn't hold on to me though she'd taken me into her heart. So the next day we went our separate ways and I roamed around a Vienna I didn't know and that didn't know me, high on the crest of a manic wave. I couldn't leave either, I kept missing trains, I spent the night in some green space, with a snack bar over there on the edge of it where a conceited Rainhard Fendrich was having a beer and joking around. And in my head the constant loop of Fendrich's song "Have You Seen Vienna by Night?" Well, I haven't yet, thanks for asking, but I'm seeing it now, my friend, and how! as I storm through it, Vienna by night, past the cathedrals, through the twisty streets, sugary, prettified, death driven, just like Malenka, just like me, so beyond and great and absolutely destructive.

After two days I managed to catch a train to Munich. I spent a night there in Malenka's apartment to which she'd returned. A short breather. Then on to Berlin. Whenever I sensed a conductor coming, I took refuge in the toilet. Once again, I didn't have the money for a ticket.

46

Lithium is not something the industry pushes, the head doctor told me on his round with the other doctors, caregivers, and psychologists. It doesn't have a lobby because it's so cheap, a salt in an alkali metal, which is known to exist in nature. This from the head doctor Anja had recommended. He didn't look at me during his explanation, spoke rapidly and without error, in well-formed, hasty sentences, all the while staring at his files.

There are reasons why patients refuse to take psychopharmaceuticals or stop taking them, lithium included. They seriously impair cognition, make it difficult to understand and remember what you have read or experienced, and slow down your mind; they make the sedated patient dull, reduce their responsiveness and blur their concentration. This results in a retreat from society, in passivity, malaise, indifference. Nothing is of interest anymore, onerous emptiness prevails. And those are only some of the negative effects on cognition caused by phase stabilizers such as lithium. Physical side effects include weight gain, nausea, hair loss, reduced libido, vertigo.

The wonderful perfidy of his explanation is worth examining: the head doctor did not tell me about the effects but about the industry. And in doing so he didn't even mention the usual suspicion that the psychopharma industry is just an enormous money-making machine that pushes useless but lucrative chemical bombshells onto the patients; this made lithium appear more trustworthy than other medications could ever be. I don't know whether he presented this argument, a kind of indie argument, to all the patients, or just to those who resisted medication. In my case, his statements confused my objections and weakened them. I was still refusing to take this lithium, which I knew mainly from a once-loved Nirvana song that mystified it too much. But he implanted an argument that was different from what I'd heard or read so far. Months later it finally took root and developed effects. I didn't know it yet, but at some point I would take lithium.

47

But first things went downhill some more. The social worker at the hospital found me a spot in a transition centre. I had to live somewhere, didn't I? Life motif: transition in transit. I wasn't yet aware that I was in a tight spot, and it would take years to work my way out of the heap of debts and the social trap I was already caught in. I was hardly even aware of the plain fact that I was now living in a transition centre. What did it matter anyway? Just a room, with dreams in it. Besides, hadn't that also happened to David Foster Wallace? Didn't George Orwell live in Paris as a tramp? And what had been going on with Helmut Krausser in those years he describes in his Hagen-the-Drinker Trilogy? And why did I need to list all these earlier cases? This was a unique experience, I just needed to take it the right way. And so I accepted everything, the porous everyday, the hectic moves, the absurd conversations, with less and less in my luggage and less of an identity in my head too. Because of a passing obsession with Charlottenburg, I landed in Berlin's west end. And became a west-end boy: *down and out at Ku'damm and Olympiastadion.*

Those were now my stomping grounds, and I combed through them every day. I visited the odious stadium, and berated the Nazis in my mind, I roamed around the Schlosspark, wandered up and down the Kaiserdamm, and recognized spots I'd explored with William T. Vollmann, went to the zoo, the Grunewald, and walked down the

Kantstrasse. I thought about the actor Frank Giering who'd lived there and drunk himself to death a few months earlier. And then, more and more often I got into the U-Bahn number 2 at Theodor-Heuss-Platz to go visit the old neighbourhoods, out of pure nostalgia. I had no clear idea of my situation, but I was temporarily making the best of it.

Music came shrilling from my headphones, drowning out my environment. I could no longer stand that every time I listened in, people's chit-chat continued to refer to me, still meant me. It was bizarre, I turned the music up so loud that people in the seats beside me complained. If I hadn't already had tinnitus, I would have developed it.

Patrick, who I ran into on the Brunnenstrasse one day with my headphones on, referred to me as Travis Bickle, from *Taxi Driver*, in a conversation he had with Aljoscha. And like a taxi driver I was constantly on the go in my Eminem wife-beater, weighed down with two jam-packed shoulder bags by Pelle Mia (please exchange the first letters), whose straps cut into my naked shoulders. My manic uniform.

Sometimes I had so little money I shook Maggi seasoning sauce down my throat just to get the taste of food in my mouth. I felt this was more of a joke than a predicament, because very soon I would be unbelievably rich, and this here, this home, the weirdos in it, the Maggi, were just one more test, to be taken with humour, before I made the great breakthrough. Then push-ups.

The mania was persistent but I was acting less driven than before. The attacks that my life of excess had unleashed against me, the ambushes and the downturns, had had some effects. In spite of the energy surges, I was damaged and weakened, I retreated, didn't want much to do with people anymore. And slowly the mountains of debt came into view. Overdue notices arrived, threats, letters from collection agencies, court decisions. I wrote back in the name of former Interior Minister Otto Schily. I would be hiring him as my lawyer, I said; he would be raising his voice against the state again as he had done at Stammheim. A letter from the lawyer Peter Raue came in too. It was an order to maintain a distance of a certain number of metres between myself and the publisher Ulla Unseld-Berkéwicz. Sure, I responded, insolently, closer contact was intolerable anyway, it was against my nature, and furthermore, in an excess of generosity I was herewith waiving the honorarium owed me for the translation of a short text by Vollmann titled "Absinthe." In the letter I also refuted Raue's academic titles, one by one, and mocked this "West Berlin dandy" right to his face, as best I could. The wit of someone in despair, who knew nothing of his own desperate condition.

My agent Robert still supported me. Twice a week, I would go by for a meal, maintaining contact to more stable people there. Whenever an email I sent to the agency was too hectic or full of mistakes, he would worry and inquire if I'd "tanked up" too much again. He began to take my finances in hand, and looked after them for two more years, especially when, in the depression that followed, the full extent of my financial ruin was revealed. Sometimes I would sit in the agency kitchen, chatter on to the women employed there, and work, if that was possible. Suddenly the novel *Sickster*, that had been years in the making, was nearing production. After the scandal with Suhrkamp I had landed with Rowohlt Berlin, which, in retrospect, was a good thing. Now I had to finish up the novel, keep the last scraps of my concentration intact, and focus. Oddly, the segments I wrote while I was manic are not the crazy, wild episodes of the novel; they are transition texts, almost filler texts, plot-movers, that I don't much like. I was writing as though on a leash.

Everything has been damaged, my life, my works. I wonder which narrative texts have not been stylistically disfigured: this book, and the novel *3000 Euros*. The plays have all more or less escaped damage—I wonder why? Because they had to be created within a few months, and not in the times when I was ill? Only hypomanic writers, lightly loony authors, can produce readable or performable material during their episodes. True manics write nothing but nonsense, and I was no exception. Most of my work has been damaged, partially beyond my control. Some of the later stories in *Raumforderung* read like accounts of my illness, which is what they are. I don't read them, I just remember them. A young psychiatrist told me that collection ought to be required reading for psychiatrists in training. I figure that is both a compliment and an expression of empathy.

Bipolar disorder has come between me and everything I ever wanted to be. It has made the life I wanted to live impossible, even if I hardly had an idea what that life might be. It has battered the books I wrote. And if anyone wants to know why this narcissistic guy can't stop raving on about his works, the answer is that the works have become my life. Because I hardly have a life beyond them. Maybe that will improve at some point, but maybe it won't.

Raumforderung opens up a whole spectrum of forms, from the classic short story to deliberately exaggerated meta-narratives to experimental craziness. When the authentic made me ill, I could no longer work out the details of this spectrum, hone the fine points, expand on the differences. I couldn't pursue what I had planned. In the future, I would like to work on classic, confident, poised narration again, with all the peculiarities, obstacles, and gaps included. I haven't been capable of that, I've had too much of a struggle with this damn complex in my life. Maybe I'll succeed one day. Entire fields of corn are waiting to burst into forests of popcorn.

48

The problem is that I am under medication. And I write under medication. That seeps into my sentences, and inundates the structure. It dams up my choice of words. I constantly come up with qualifiers such as "more or less," "maybe," "perhaps," "a kind of," for fear of excessive feeling, and maybe for lack of it too, out of the need to cook things on the backburner. The medication lops off the apexes, as they say, the high ones and the low ones, in life and in writing. This brings on a new sobriety, sets up a resistance I have to overcome in order to express anything. And the medicine has its grip on every last nerve fibre. *That* is my syntax, Dr Benn.

Further, each episode of the illness destroys brain mass, as British researchers have discovered. It has not yet been established if stress-related hormones or genetic dispositions are responsible. But it has been proven that in bouts of the illness the brain shrinks in volume and the more numerous the attacks that test subjects have suffered the lower the scores they earn in IQ and language testing. The bouts massively destroy nerve cells and neuronal networks.

What does this mean? I don't know. Is it just the process of aging that makes me a calmer, less shrill storyteller? Is it just the medication that hems me in and controls me? Is it both, inextricably entangled? And how am I meant to relate to it all? This has become the exact opposite of the booze-and-drugs writers who whip up unleashed-word excess; this is sedation speaking. It is sloth taking control of my body and stopping my words from flipping out. Is that a good thing? Is it a bad thing? If ever I forget to take my medication in the evening, or deliberately don't take it, I feel a different strength in me the next day. Even if I only imagine this effect, it is still there. And on the other hand, if I notice, when I'm on the phone, that I'm talking too fast again and getting ahead of myself, or if I catch myself pacing back and forth in my apartment too hectically, I immediately drop a special med. Then I slam those pills down my throat with such voracious force it scares me.

It's actually about survival. Without this pacification, without the destruction of these neuronal networks, I would no longer exist. The medication is saving my life. But at what price?

49

I am stretched out in the bathtub, feeling agitated from writing, worried and afraid that what I am doing might be wrong, an error, a dead-end, *the* end—and then, suspended in these loops, I am seized by the fear, reaching right into my body, of going manic again, losing everything again, right here, right now. My thoughts grow hectic, sentence fragments get stuck in my head, there is movement in the windings of my brain, perceptible, involuntary, that's how it starts, isn't it? I've actually forgotten how it starts. My heart is racing. Then I see the images from the PET scans of my brain light up above me, in vivo and in colour, showing the different regions transforming and changing colour. Places that were usually asleep in cool blue are now bursting into garish colour like in CNN reports on bomb attacks, yellow and red and bright orange. My breathing becomes panting. "Quiet," I whisper to myself, which echoes in the empty bathroom, "quiet, quiet, quiet, quiet, quiet."

50

Fatigued, I look up from the medical textbooks: classifi-
cations, renamings, new categorizations, different rubrics,
statistics. What good does it do me to know what the
hypotheses are about disturbances in transmitter systems,
or what blood values allow conclusions about certain noradrenalin distribution, and where in the limbic system
there may have been cellular stress or neurotrophic stasis
before the collapse?

I cannot know, because they don't know. They simply
do not know how it works, this disease, the medication,
they're feeling their way in the dark, with just a few glimmers of light, but the closer you come the more diffuse and
weak they become. The statistics, too, constantly produce
contradictory, new, and immediately out-of-date results
while the numbers provided by the studies never match.
How many percent exactly? If a fact arrives, it is just a
temporary indicator. Goddamn blood-brain barrier! I will
never find myself in these texts.

Nor can I find comfort, as many others do, in references
to manic-depressive artists in the past. Ellen Forney, for
instance, a comic-artist who read Kay Redfield Jamison's
book *Touched with Fire* as I did, a book that thematizes the
connection between bipolar disorder and creativity, is herself manic-depressive. She extracts an uncanny comfort
from this book and calls Melville, Woolf, Henry James,
Poe, Strindberg part of her inner circle. For me, nothing is
more unlikely. The problems we have in life are not even
touched upon by drawing parallels to great writers. And as
I've said before I have no conceits about this illness; on the
contrary, it fills me with distress, alienation, and shame.

"Can you channel that?" somebody asks, who claims to
be like me. He is dead drunk and making a lot of noise. He

seems to be proud of his diagnosis; it serves to legitimize his role as an overbearingly stupid bigmouth and doesn't trigger even a vague shimmer of a thought in him. He is not sick, but he is celebrating the findings. All you need to do is channel it, he yells with a meaningful look at me, in a parallel condition. Then, in the nagging voice of a dictator no one can take seriously, he yells across the room at the servers. Another bottle of red wine. All you need to do is channel it, he says again.

Do it with pride, another acquaintance says, if you do it, do it with pride. And in fact, this back and forth between pride and shame is one of the central movements in my life, like the flittering between megalomania and minority complexes. But I can't just do "it" "with pride." That would be a rapper pose, the histrionics of a poseur. That would be Bukowski. I keep getting compared to him anyway. I have to do it differently.

Nor do I believe in madness being some kind of blessing, as Socrates suggests in *Phaedrus*, or in the godlike "art of mad prophecy," which is Schleiermacher's punning translation of mania in Plato's text. Madness is not a gift of prophecy. I detest the pseudo-archetypal images that Hollywood produces under the idiotic label of "the mad genius"; the film industry has contributed massively to the demonization but also the glorification of psychic defects. And when a manic-depressive character like Carrie Mathison in *Homeland* appears, that character ends up immediately neutralizing an entire commando of terrorists, face twisted into an intensely seething expression but never doing anything really crazy in their manic bouts. In films and TV series, manic-depressives are either shown as viciously dangerous crazies who slash their way through life, or as highly talented genius loners whose talents have unfortunately distended into disease—or a third option, which is all the more desirable because it fires up the horror: they are both. Movie characters who are psychically ill are often criminals whose obsession drives them to ever more brutal actions; they cannot help but present their twisted image to the world around them, do violence to the norm that has let them slip down into this illness. Of course, the abnormal always throws the normal into relief, which is often already sick enough. But for the purposes of dramaturgy and sensationalism, the abnormal is generally simplified and trivialized.

In reality, people who are mad are usually victims who are no longer able to find their way in life, who end up hospitalized or homeless or lurch through the streets as tangled bundles of nerves where they may suffer rape or murder; they themselves only rarely commit rape or murder. Or they are average, neither highly talented nor disabled people, who are sick and just have to struggle with their sickness. It is not all an "abyss." People just like horror.

And even though a disproportionate number of writers and artists seem to suffer from bipolar disorder, I would gladly cancel my membership in this illustrious club, with immediate effect. The disease may indeed have some positive aspects for certain individuals, for those who are artistically inclined, and the driven single-mindedness that comes with hypomania can produce valuable results and nurture the avant-garde, but I would still gladly cancel my membership and make that retroactive—even though Kay Jamison claims that artists and manics think on a broader scale, moving spontaneously back and forth across it. The creative act always involves a regression to more primitive levels of the mental hierarchy for which a mild mania can offer a functional structure while other processes continue to operate in a more rational place. I would still slam the door so hard the entire structure would collapse.

The illness may be destructive for the individual who suffers from it, but according to a recent insight it can offer advantages to society. Not only artists, but also a sizable proportion of exceptional minds in science, politics, and economics are afflicted by milder forms of the disease. If such a thing as social progress occurs, it is driven by these people. Ironically, even the Nazis, who murdered or forcibly sterilized tens of thousands of my kind in their eugenic cleansing programs, had to admit that the effects of manic-depressive illness can have certain advantageous social aspects. In a study done in the 1930s, Hans Luxenburger, a psychiatrist and "racial hygienist," declares that the disease is over-represented in higher-level and academic social classes, which is why he advises against the sterilization of these patients, especially if the patient in question does not have siblings who could pass on the positive aspects of this inheritance. An American study from the early 1940s (and the Americans were pioneers in eugenics in the early twentieth century) addresses the same topic of the proportion of bipolar patients in "socially successful" circles, and comes to a similar conclusion. Formulated in more flowery language, the study claims that if it were possible to eliminate those who are ill with manic-depressive psychoses and remove them from this world, we would deprive ourselves of an "immeasurable wealth of capability and talent, of colour and warmth of spirit, of innovation."

Others, however, say it's just our heritage from the Neanderthals.

51

Then I meet a Finnish woman in a bar, and over the many hours of conversation she challenges my thinking in her robot-like English, my thinking about myself, about the disease, about my position in the world and in society. She can hear the self-flagellation in my words. She resists it, in a strange kind of way, but without any esoteric posturing. So why do I think I have to conform even more after going through all that suffering? Why do I assume that everything I believed then is wrong? Why do I think I need to rein in my anger? And why do I not make even more stringent demands for the right to insist on my way of being, my existence?

If she were to read this book, she might understand. But still, we spend almost an entire day talking this through, to and fro and fro and to. I have never had a more dogged advocate. In the end those few hours were actually good for me.

Of course, there is another, "better" side to the illness. You can speak of the personal profundity it adds to your life, your thinking, your feeling, or of an existential resonance, which, if deprived of these experiences, might never be accessible. By crossing the boundaries of my feelings and thoughts, I have taken their measure, come into contact with the outskirts of existence and preparations for the afterlife of the human, whose existence and qualities I could only surmise. I know my abyss, I know my demons. It is absurd that some people envy you that, are envious that you *even have* a fate, or would themselves really like to "go off the deep end sometime," leave everything behind, "like you." Occasionally I hear things from an overly analyzed perspective that suggests I may proactively have *entered* the manic bouts, deliberately sought them out. That is absolutely groundless, especially in view of all the disasters, but it shows how much ignorance the patient has to face, even on the part of people who are familiar with psychic defects. And even the patients themselves don't always see clearly:

sedated, reintegrated, and slogging through the grey every-day, some of them yearn for the intensity the illness once triggered in them. All I can say is I now know things I never would have known; I have access to an intuitive treasure trove of knowledge. I know that my own suffering has strengthened and refined the empathy I feel for others. The illness has taken me places that were terrifying and revelatory at once, and I now know the entire spectrum of the society in which I live; I may also be more sensitive to the repressions this society enacts because I have suffered them. The illness may have broken me forever. But maybe, and against my will, it also made me a writer.

52

I remember hauling a shopping cart laden with my tele-vision and other stuff, books and especially cables along the sidewalk in front of the International Congress Cen-tre. (I still own the TV and the cables.) I get angry, maybe because it's such a stupid thing to be doing, maybe because of my pointless action, and I shove it along ahead of me with jerks and jolts. It clatters dramatically, rattles over the asphalt in great arcs, and almost tips over. Motorists are thinking their thoughts. They can do that. They're welcome to witness my cranky anger as they go by. I do *not* wave at them. Most of my things are still in storage in the container. I hate the container. Bertram says the build-ing with the containers could make a really good set for a detective movie, for a murder, for instance. Right on, I say, with the voice of a curmudgeonly commissar.

I no longer know where I live. Everything is in pieces. I heave the shopping cart into the S-Bahn. It almost doesn't work, one wheel gets jammed in the gap between the train and the platform. Then I yank it in, with one power-jerk that

makes a stab of pain shoot down my back. I reap the irritated glances of the other passengers with the pride of a leper.

I remember the countless cables I buy. At some point
they end up in an immense tangled mess in my room, a
veritable sea monster that keeps growing in menace and
that can't be sorted, especially not by fumbling hands.
Later I will consider misusing one of the cables.

I remember Sonja, my social worker, the only person
who can still calm me down. She's from Hamburg and I
love her dry but still warm-hearted ways. When I get a
bloody cut in my forehead from smashing it into the wash
basin, actually breaking the wash basin with my forehead,
she realizes that I must be having another bout. I question
this. She doesn't realize that I've been manic all along. I am
really good at dissimulating. She takes me to the hospital
where they sew up the wound. Never before have I seen
as much blood as there was on the white tiles in my room.

I remember Max, the gnome. He was abused as a child, I
am not sure if that included sexual abuse. He has a hunch-
back. A hundred times a day he yells, "Shit" down the corridor. If you ask him a question he answers quietly and calmly.

I remember the guy whose shed I damaged grinning at
me in a bar and making a snide remark that I'd now evidently arrived at the very bottom rung of the social ladder.
I wonder why that was so gratifying for him.

I remember banishing all that into a fictional text titled
3000 Euros and how I managed to do this only by fiction-
alizing it all in passages that have nothing to do with what
actually happened.

There is so much I don't remember, but I do remember the
professor, much later, who wrote an assessment in which he
claimed that manics remember everything. He is blatantly
wrong. His whole career is herewith damned and doomed.

I remember my mother's constant faxes, the warnings and notices she sent on, labelled in fat, meaningless script—meant for my TO-DO LIST—as though that would change anything. And on the side, her little greetings, a sun and clouds, laughing and crying.

I remember having two laptops stolen, one in a café because I went to the washroom and thought nothing would happen, there were good spirits watching over me, and the other in the S-Bahn because I fell asleep, exhausted. They took my entire bag. I remember being lured into a trap after I got into a fight with a supposed terrorist in the Rote Rose (Red Rose) Bar, a place for down-and-outs that, according to the musician Wolfgang Müller, counted the playwright Heiner Müller as one of its eternal visitors. We'll go outside, the supposed terrorist said, and I thought, okay; I followed him, an accomplice tripped me up as we were heading out, I stumbled, another accomplice grabbed my wallet from my pants pocket and ran off with it. You can't tell them apart, the policewoman said.

I remember the madness of four prostitutes at the same time, from the back and the front, and two days later meeting one of them again at a traffic light, and her winking and laughing at me.

I remember a night somewhere in Prenzlauer Berg when I get lost in the snow and can't find my way back, completely exhausted and tired. At that point I am too frightened to ask anyone for directions—directions to where, anyway? And why am I so frightened? Wherever I go I hear hissed messages, garish slogans, fake news, and madly ticking telex machines. Depending on my perspective that day, I see the media as a great big gift or as a monumental horror, as total torture. At the moment, everything is torture.

Besides, that night someone threatened me with a set of

brass knuckles. I'd been on the go for days, without direction, or meaning, or purpose, and was sitting there in the
S-Bahn, completely wiped out, when two young guys came
up. For some reason, one of them held his knuckle-duster
in my face. The other passengers moved away from us, got
up from their seats. I kept the two guys at bay with talk,
stormed out at the next stop, into a wind-tossed Grunewald,
ran on and on until I was able to slow down because they
weren't following me any longer. The music of Tegan
and Sara was on my MP3 player. There was an incredible
windstorm that night, trees and branches were pitching
and plunging in all directions, the night was alive. I wandered on for hours, through the woods, through the storm,
because I didn't dare go back to the S-Bahn where the guys
with the brass knuckles who I had in no way threatened, no
way at all, would doubtless find me and beat me up. What
was up with them? What "sister" were they talking about?
Man! People are crazy, and the police have nothing to say
about it. They've constantly got their eye on me, but when
I'm in danger they don't take it seriously. The world has
turned on me. Who can I turn to? There's nobody around
anyway. The cold is cutting into me.

 I don't know where I am, it seems I've walked around
in the same circle three times. I'm not wearing enough
clothing either, shivering, no longer shivering, just gone
rigid. My internal energy can't keep me warm anymore.
And there's black ice all over the place. Claus Peymann,
the artistic director of the Berliner Ensemble, got excited
about the city not salting the courtyard there; on TV he
reported people slipping and falling in front of his theatre,
yet another scandal, unacceptable, and in typical Peymann
style he attacked the city managers. Now I keep slipping
and falling, here in the middle of nowhere, somewhere

among all these apartment blocks, and I keep getting up. My jeans have a dark stain on them. It hurts, I've got a cut on my shin. Where to? Finally, I find refuge in a ground-floor apartment that is under renovation. The door was ajar and I'm in a dark room with paint buckets and two ladders. How did I find this place? I don't remember, even now. Did I just walk in? I sit down on a chair in the middle of the rubble from the construction work, among tools and empty pop bottles, am immediately covered in white dust particles, and fall into a daze. It is hardly any warmer inside than it is outside. Everything is pallid and stiff.

53

I do remember the next move. Sonja had got me another apartment, in another institution, months later, just to get me out of the transition centre. I was getting physically sick there and had to constantly watch out for the two guys who pretended to be bros on the one hand but regularly cleared out other people's rooms using the keys they'd stolen from one of the caregivers. I was ready for the move. It required countless trips to offices, countless applications, to end up, once again in the care of some institution, and a bunch of new caregivers and new rules. An apartment of my own was still a long way off, I had no money, only debts and a credit rating that stank to high heaven.

We drove from west to east, over causeways and down tree-lined streets and I could feel I was heading in the right direction, in Sonja's Fiat with a few of my things in the trunk. But the new place, run by an association that fights addictions, was not right for me either, as I soon found out. They had no experience of manic depression. There was no right place for me. But I figured it didn't matter; no, I figured it's all for the best: I don't really want to be cared for,

I just want my own "living unit." And that was what I now had. It was in Kreuzberg and consisted of one small room with a kitchenette and a toilet. It was a first step. I would have to put up with the unsuitable caregivers for a while, and they would irritate me and I would curse them—but it was a first step back into what was a superficially cobbled-together life.

A life that was already beleaguered and besieged. The piles of files kept growing: reintegration procedures, debt deferrals, contracts for deliverables, case management reports, applications for support, waivers of confidentiality, reports on caregiving processes, applications to reactivate caregiving processes, confirmations of cost coverage, judicial claims enforcements, writs of execution. A neurologist's expert opinion said it was a case of manic-depressive psychosis, with currently hypomanic manifestations due to abated mania (ICD 10 F31.1) as well as chronic alcohol abuse (ICD 10 F10.1). There was insufficient information on treatment, no medication at the moment, and I was incapable of managing my affairs in regard to "finances, health care, assisted living facilities, contact with government agencies, courts of law, or housing associations." The illness was chronic, there was evidence of a seriously impaired capacity for self-care. Without care I would be unable to develop sufficiently rational insights about my health, and I had an insufficient understanding of my personal affairs.

Oral communication with me might be possible.

54

Kreuzberg, this utopia we were inhabiting, that we'd created, how brightly it was gleaming this spring day! I roamed through the neighbourhood I'd assimilated into years earlier, quite naturally, instinctively, unaware of the fate that linked us. Already dizzy, I hurried through Görlitzer Park, over bridges and down pathways that felt like clockwork to me, and were apparently overtaking time. A small heading in the *Frankfurter Allgemeine Zeitung* had set off this image of the city as clockwork, and now I was experiencing it. Then I read out the street names posted everywhere for the people's orientation, and felt happy about them. How diverse were their uses and how lovely their sounds.

Everything made sense. I now had a much better retroactive understanding of social and private encounters. Clearly that man had said what he said to protect us from the truth, and that argument had developed because the situation was so complex and crazy nobody could understand it let alone express it.

I was at peace with everything. Even the most involved connections glowed in a different light, in this springtime light, gleaming and fresh and new. From this angle, my screwed-up childhood was understandable. I forgave everyone and was happy. We had just managed to avoid catastrophe; it was over now, utopia was drawing near, paradisal conditions would reign supreme. And the Kreuzberg light gently dimmed, shining softly in all directions, and back again.

55

That was spring 2011. So I was still crazy. The mania had been going on for over a year. It had settled in, was no longer in question, I no longer cared if I was the messiah. My paranoid view of the world was the norm and at the same time transparent, a thin layer over everything I perceived, but it no longer played a big role. Like a plastic film, it stuck to everything I felt and thought.

The illness subsided slowly, but it did subside. We were both tired of each other, exhausted. Occasionally it would rear up again and I would join in, which resulted in a few side-view mirrors broken off cars, for which I went to court and paid fines. Or a rather strange birthday binge I set up in a restaurant, with strangers but also old friends who came by and eyed me skeptically, among them Aljoscha. Sometimes I would fire up my mood with alcohol, leap up, and start berating the absent Nick Cave at a PJ Harvey concert, but these were brief episodes, hardly worth mentioning. For a few days I planted myself in the Rheinische Vertretung (Rhineland Representation) restaurant on Friedrichstrasse, occupied the smoking cabin, worked there with my ersatz laptop in front of me. I hissed, "Shame on you!" at Günter Grass, who actually turned up one day. I bought a shit-yellow leather jacket, threw it in the washing machine, sprayed blue splotches all over it, shredded it into bluish-yellow tatters that hung on my body and wandered about the streets in it, feeling overheated and proud. But the paths I took were shorter, my attacks of fury were shorter. The waves were decreasing in number and flattening out. It could be only a matter of weeks until I broke down. The lithium would speed up this process.

56

Ella had entered my life, and I really liked her, I'd even fallen in love. I still wonder today what it was she liked about a manic. She seemed to have spotted something there, something worth keeping and loving despite the trouble that I still, occasionally, caused.

I started taking the lithium because Ella asked me to. Robert had asked me as well. Aljoscha had been asking forever, and my new doctor, whose bourgeois Bavarian semi-pomposity made him more acceptable than most of the other doctors I'd had, urged it on me. And the statements of the head doctor at St. Hedwig Hospital were having their effect too; nobody earns much with this stuff, I told myself, citing him, it's a salt, it's natural, I told myself, it is sidelined by the pharmaceutical industry. So I finally picked some up and took it for the first time in the little kitchenette in my apartment. I remember how I imagined I could feel it working on my brain mere moments later, a light tingling sensation just below the top of my skull. I walked down to the Admiral Bridge, tingling as I went, and thought now everything will be fine.

The bridge had long been our meeting place. When I was in treatment that was where I would meet with Aljoscha, Knut, and Patrick, Friday nights in spring 2007, have a smoke and half a beer with them, hops on my tongue a mark of freedom, and then shuffle the three hundred metres back to the hospital and check back in. Later, once I was more or less back in order, we'd kept this meeting spot until it became so full of tourists and buskers that we gave it up.

Now I was sitting there alone on one of the pilings, gazing at the friendly glimmer in the sky and actually thinking, it'll be good again. A lightness seemed to return to my head.

And it actually was good again, but differently than I expected. Within days the mad constructs that I'd dragged with me for almost a year and a half and that had long turned brittle, collapsed in a cloud of dust and the hypertrophic feelings finally died away. Suddenly, the apartment was a normal apartment, men were men, women were women, and a poem was damn well a poem. The zillion layers that everything and everyone had displayed, disappeared; what remained was a single, smooth, innuendo-free surface, the simplest and most obvious of all realities, sheer material. An enormous fatigue overcame me and emotions submerged in deafness.

For a start people didn't know me anymore. They looked away, not deliberately, not under duress, they just did. They followed their own thoughts, along random or regular pathways, in couples, as passersby, lover-less or just as loners on bridges and in parks, and our eyes did not meet unless I insisted. Humanity was no longer focused on me. That was a relief, but also an irritant. They all seemed to simply pass me by in normal self-absorption. That had not been my experience in a long time. But I still pushed this perception aside, the paranoia had riled me up for too long and too insistently. In fact, I didn't really push it aside, it's just that paranoia was playing less and less of a role. I could sense something changing but didn't let that seep further into my thoughts or harden into recognition. My persecution complex died away without me being conscious of it. It just happened, that's how it was, and my head was pounding. Those were the days of the dawning.

I also began to realize that some of the judgements I'd made and lived through were simply not true. The question, "Did you go crazy again?" crept into the blurred lines of my thought but remained unanswered. The process was sluggish, not one of instantaneous insight. And my feelings were also in a twilight zone. I grew more and more fatigued. Slept whenever I could. Thought little.

The suspicion that my thinking over the last months, over the entire last year had been tainted with madness and been simply wrong, became more and more of a certainty, but I didn't yet realize it fully. This wasn't right, and that wasn't either. What had I been thinking? I'd already forgotten. I forgot it all over again and lay down. So much wasn't right. Everything was falling apart.

In case the reader is now sighing deeply and thinking, oh no, not again, not another downward spiral into depression, may this reassure the reader: the person living this story felt the same way.

It was like one of those blows to the head in a comic strip. The victim, lying in a corner with stars whirling around his head, his groggy eyes fixed on empty space, is trying to collect himself. He slowly finds his way back, his thoughts accompany him in fragments, and after the blow to the head there is often a new insight—which leads him into madness, into genius, or back to normalcy. The slow whirl of stars in my head led me back to normality, but it hit me like a shock.

My obsession with celebrities stuck around for a short manic moment, I remember that. Trent Reznor won an Oscar for the soundtrack of *The Social Network*, and when he made his thank-you speech I read his lips and understood that he was obviously dedicating it to me. Standing in the dark kitchenette I thought about this. I can't believe it, I thought, he's still on my side. I've lost everything but he's still on my side. He's dedicated his prize to me. We would soon be working together. Oh, yeah.

57

And then, of course, the TRENT OBSESSION that will also be part of the novel. Nine Inch Nails is the only band that has stayed with me, intact, through two psychoses, and accompanied me since 1995. It's a prole band, it's dreadful, it's bipolar, it's brilliant, it's loud, it's furious, it's addicted, it's embarrassing, it's childish, it's tender. It's dangerous, it's full of hate, it's against love, it's wounded, but it's everything but loveless, it's everything but only wounded, it displays its wound, it screams out its hatred and always ends up turning on itself, it's dark, it's garish, it's inspired, it's primitive, it's sick, and it's great—it has spoken to me for the last fifteen years. In the snobbish environs of the arrogant meta-metastifying stylist, Nabokov was always floating somewhere overhead, as someone outside had already remarked, while in the actual desperation of life Trent Reznor was always there behind me. It's dark, but it's so dark that the only lightness is in true darkness, ghostlike, phosphorescently glowing, perhaps greenish but definitely a paler shimmer, the only one that lasts, the last one remaining. I can only read Nabokov when I feel good; I can only listen to Trent Reznor when I feel bad. The reasons will be researched; no, not researched they will be PRESENTED; something like that. Because they play a prominent role in the novel, the protagonist is a NIN fan, what a coincidence. He like me, me not like him, he already like him, me not yet like me.

(Part of a blog post, January 5, 2010)

58

I stood there, gazed at the dark shelf with the two plates, and paused. What? But yeah. Trent had stood there in his tuxedo with the golden statue in his hand and muttered the dedication into the applause. Yes, that was exactly how it was. I threw myself on my bed.

Sure. This collaboration would take place. Nine Inch Nails and me, gleaming black dystopias, soul terror, and technoid turmoil against the structural depressions in the entire apparatus of flesh.

It took just a minute until this fantasy, too, dissipated. He dedicated the Oscar to me? He did not. What nonsense, how did I ever get there? He didn't even know me. How embarrassing.

The last bits were gone. I got up and looked around. It became clear to me that everything, really everything I'd thought over the past months, was completely wrong and wacky, a wild and multifaceted fabulation, a monster in my head. How could I have thought all that? I tried to suppress it, because I'd suddenly also became aware of my behaviour, and the consequences of my behaviour, and the consequences of the consequences, all of which sent me reeling into a panic.

I looked around this unfamiliar, drab room that had hardly any furniture. A cupboard, a mattress. A few boxes over there with stuff inside that the hostile temporary sublet a few months earlier had contemptuously referred to as "garbage," and that was ever more reduced, more randomized. The kitchenette over there, small and ugly, next to it the glum little stub of a corridor with the messy files. Where had I ended up? What did I still have?

I sat down on the big, threadbare office chair, took a breath, and held it. That would become a new tic: holding my breath, maintaining the tension in my swelling body, approaching death. Holding my breath, again and again, consciously at first, soon unconsciously, automatically, even as I write, until I finish the sentence.

The back courtyard outside, yet another of these damn back courtyards in this hostile city, one of the infamous Berlin back courtyards that scan by me like on some senseless search screen.

Breath, held in, perpetuated. Silence.

59

The anchors of my existence had been torn away, swept away. I had no bank account, no apartment of my own, only debts and court cases to deal with. I was in a halfway house, officially homeless and "mentally disabled." That was what a clear look at the situation revealed, a look not veiled or smeared with madness, that's how it was, objectively.

I had arrived where I'd never been before: in a hole of an "assisted living" room that was functional and unfurnished, with the marks earlier tenants had left, stickers on the fridge, dents in the walls: pushed to the very edge. The sheets I put on the bed had holes in them. I'd hung jackets and hoodies over the smeared, curtainless windows. I sat down and had a smoke.

When I say I was pushed, that's not correct, because my situation was, of course, caused by me. This was the result of my actions. But I still felt harassed by the system, excluded from life, prosecuted and sanctioned by the state. What was labelled "help" in the following months would be automatized management without any real prospect of reintegration. I looked in the fridge. The light worked, stains of mysterious origin had dried onto the bottom shelf. I debated what I should buy in order to stock it. I couldn't think of anything except milk, cheese, and butter. I succeeded in shutting the fridge door on the third try, everything was worn out, and I left the apartment in order to get to know the neighbourhood at a slower pace.

It's almost like war. A pretentious, almost obscene comparison but it's true: as a temporarily cured madman I was now a sort of war casualty, bombed out of my house, driven into exile and homelessness, robbed and deprived of everything I owned; internally also deprived of all my property because most of what I'd loved and read had been contaminated by the radiation of madness. Madness is a destructive war inside yourself, that's obvious, and the seriously afflicted may experience this war several times in their lives and salvage less and less each time.

60

The grief that now overcame me was bleaker and more austere than before. I had seen it all before in weaker form, a déjà vu of horror. At the same time the grief burrowed into me so subtly that we became one. It accompanied everything I did. I was virtually paralyzed for those weeks and months, but I carried on, somehow. The last remaining people around me breathed sighs of relief: he was finally quiet. But the depression pulled me down, along with the certainty that I had ruined my life forever.

This grief is still a part of me today. It has tinged my life, though there are nuances, sometime a deep darkness that lets pass no word or glance, sometimes just a grey filter that veils everything but that I can almost ignore if I just focus on the colours. Maybe one day I will be rid of this grief. Maybe, *once*, time will be on my side.

And considering the extent of the disaster I'm surprised I managed without further hospital stays or suicide attempts.

61

That was thanks to Ella. She kept me afloat in those weeks and months, without any fuss. She'd come by with "kids' food": fish sticks, potatoes, and vegetables, leftovers from her daughters' meals—or we'd go to the movies. Or we'd just sit on her couch talking or watching a TV series or reading something to each other, then drive through the city, have breakfast, and go for a walk at the Schlachtensee. What may sound like boring normality here was a kind of wonder. Because normality was about as far removed from me as you can imagine. Blackness and bleakness were all around. But Ella supported me, kept me upright. She seemed to see a person who was not yet there, or no longer there. He was not yet present—not as the hotspur she'd met or the abject weakling I was about to become. Or maybe he was, but only in silhouette in the occasional gesture. At least for Ella.

It is easier to write about it than it was to live it. It was a difficult time. My brain tries to block it out whenever it can. Andrea Breth, the theatre director who also suffers from the classic and most crushing form of this illness, said in an interview that you have to objectify what you remember (she's referring to the manic condition, but this applies to the depression as well), because otherwise you cannot deal with it. Once I finish this book I will have to do that again too. My consciousness has to close off and shut away those phases of my present, wherever possible, if possible.

My mood grew darker, taking on ever deeper hues. You'd think black is black, but no, black can become even blacker. The cables came back into view. If Ella had abandoned me at that point, I don't know what would have happened. It is such a horror you can scarcely envision it, an unwanted form of blackmail that comes out of the blue without anyone willing it, inhumane in and of itself. She countered this burden by reading the medical literature on the web and gathering information on lithium. A theoretical framework can help, but it cannot overcome the actual symptoms or the sad little heap of misery lying there.

And then there was the night we drove to a local help centre to talk to someone, anyone from outside who might be able to advise, might offer a little comfort. Of course, the counsellor on duty we talked to was overworked in the most clichéd way. And did she really have her hair in a perm, an upside-down poodle on her head that jittered to the rhythm of her words? I was so tired of it all. I'd run out of patience, with myself, with others, but still I needed to let time go by. I knew far more about this illness than the people in these official help centres. What could they possibly tell me? Still, just having driven this distance brought on a little hope and was a sign: the two of us, bonding, for the two of us, together.

It was an attempt at love that, besides the usual squabbles, which soon increased in vehemence, also had to deal with the issue that one of the lovers was a burden on himself and on others, a weight that pulled everything down, hung there limp and heavy, not even swaying, and would really have liked to be torn off by some unknown hand and discarded. I stuck it out with Ella, who stuck it out with me while I tolerated her even when she could no longer tolerate me. And in the process, paradoxically, the loveliest moments emerged.

The lithium unfortunately gave me a pretty acute case of acne that spread across my face and my back and settled in there. This potential side effect of the salt occurs only rarely, as the literature says, but it does occur—so why not in my case? Every glance in the mirror was unexpectedly colourful. For months I went around covered in pimples and boils, gaining weight in the process and losing more and more of the hair on my head. It was hard to concentrate. When I received an award in Paris, Ella covered up the acne with makeup before the ceremony. The ceremony was awful. It appears, from the account on the internet, that I gave a speech, which I don't remember. The ministers of culture of the two nations stood beside me, and I performed whatever it was I thought I had to perform. The wine came just at the right moment, and I guzzled it. Only the meal with Ella in a restaurant at the Odéon made up for the stress, and the beauty of Paris was restored although a few hours earlier I'd walked the streets in tears.

I finally had to change the medication as the first small scars were developing and the acne wasn't subsiding. I slackened off on the lithium and took valproic acid instead, a medication for epilepsy. I am taking it to this day.

After a particularly disastrous evening—on the way home from a party Ella tore the shirt I was wearing to shreds in a rage and then insisted I spend the night with her—I wet the bed, drunk, and not yet in tune with the medication. That had never happened before. What a humiliation of nature, of medicine. Noisy protests the next morning.

Ella was pretty tenacious in her rescue efforts. I owed her but it was problematic to pay back these emotional debts, if you could even see them that way. If I gave her too much, she threw it out, if I gave her too little, she demanded everything. We'd basically become codependent in an incestuous-sibling way. She had two daughters from an earlier relationship and they kept taking potshots at the organic growth of our relationship over time; they rejected me because I didn't get involved with them. I was a child myself, a completely overbred child, tired of life, whose personality had been seriously impaired by a psychic illness. We were codependent and together only on standby.

Time weighed heavily on my soul, especially the past and the future, less so the present. We could just about handle the present, act it out, fill it. If an evening had been even partway pleasant, I thought of it as an event as I biked home, took it with me into my pillows, and used it to dull the pain. The moment was always new, always our own, and sometimes had something very liberating about it. Even a laugh could open a new path and be called into question. Because Ella had a sense of humour, spontaneous, self-deprecating, wonderfully parodic and witty. Even in my deepest misery, she could make me smile if she wanted to. And if she didn't want to, that was okay too.

I sensed that she cried more often than I did, secretly, not telling me. I rarely cried, but when I did I was the old clown without a circus again, with all the makeup that got on his face, and even under his skin, running off. Later, we'd laugh and go to the movies, and maybe to bed together. We loved each other in fact.

Ella had the hope that someday I would become a complete person again. That all this was just temporary, a task we would master, a transition. We would just have to wait long enough and be patient until a new and good life became possible. Until we could become a complete couple, consisting of two complete people, with a future.

I may have disappointed this hope. I don't know. We separated later, for other reasons, or maybe also for this reason, who can explain these things exactly? But it had been three years, and if you can tolerate pathos this time could be called a lifesaver.

62

Hey! Everything is not okay. The late-night shops, the paths leading there. The dreariness of those stores, my home, mimicry in grey. The paths leading to Ella and back, the only reason for living, hidden and not really a reason, merely an instinct, slogging through the dirt and the damp, just because it's possible. The neon signs over there that I can now decipher without seeing ten hints pointing to a hundred more connections. The new, childhood taste for sweets, every day, reaching for artificial-coloured fruit gums, actually not even fruit gums but Smurfs, that's what they were, tough blue chemistry. But whatever works: Haribo for two weeks, toasted almonds for two days, heaps of ice cream in the summer, an occasional drunk, lots of grease. The letters from the collection agencies and the courts, the debts. My growing dislike for the question about how you're doing. My aversion to sex, aversion to texts. The euphoria in the songs of Animal Collective lost to me forever. But still, growing stability and continuity in spite of and in the face of a void. My resistance to contact with others that I keep having to overcome. But things are working, most of the time.

The debts. There was pressure from all sides, every stupid subscription to a newspaper turned into months of compounding threatening letters. I wrote a short piece for *Die Zeit*, and at the same time *Die Zeit* harassed me with collection agencies. The earnings I quickly made and quickly spent exacerbated the growing debts. It reminded me of a summer job I'd had as a seventeen-year-old, working on the production line for the candy-maker Haribo, where threads of black licorice were rolled up into snail shapes. This deadly boring, tedious job would suddenly be livened up by inexplicable moments of total chaos. One of the spools might have had a speck of dirt on it, which caused a sudden wiggling heaping licorice monster to coalesce, its shiny black tentacles flailing around in a turmoil from the gyration and as soon as you managed to aim the threads into the bucket below so you could clean the spool (the licorice would flow on and fill the bucket), you'd see that all the other machines were growing the same licorice monsters, dancing around like unruly tumbleweed or excited Puli dogs, hurray, hurray, that's not the way, is what they'd be happily shouting everywhere, what the hell was going on! It must be a change in the consistency of the licorice, I said, rushing back and forth. Extreme frenzied action was the only way to clear up the shambles. Once the sixteen spools were calmly spewing out the disgusting licorice snails again, you could actually appreciate the tedium. Then boredom was a joy and it didn't matter that the smell of licorice had permeated your skin and wouldn't wash off.

Such were the debt monsters growing up around me, hurray, hurray, they yelled, that's not the way, we're here, we're growing, we're flailing about. If I managed to put down one of them, the next ones would cheerily come zigzagging over. Controlling the Haribo monsters took about half an hour; it took years to get these debts under control. And they didn't actually yell, those debt monsters, they emitted a silent terror, those thousands of letters and court orders made not a noise as they slowly throttled me. It can be managed, however; I know that today. It is possible.

These times automatically spin away from me. My consciousness cannot integrate it all. The same goes for the time I spent in the halfway house; it was obviously another person living there, though I share his memories. He's like the main character in a television series, a character I can particularly identify with.

63

Discretion makes me shy away from writing about further privacies that might involve other people and not just me. But there is this: Aljoscha became a good friend again. We managed to become closer, each in his own way. In spite of all the complications in our relationship, all the imbalances, the tensions, conflicts that any decades-long friendship might carry even without the trials ours had seen, he'd always been on my side, somewhere deep down, maybe even unwittingly. Shaken up by a fateful incident in his own family, that was different but comparable, he knew the logic of such catastrophes. We are no longer what we were, but we are present.

And I am glad of that.

64

The months passed. I dragged along after them. My status was hammered into place: sick, sick, dependent, sick. I translated novels, was numb and disciplined about it, I met the deadlines, I walked around the block, went home, headed off on the bike I'd bought on eBay, a real pile of junk, maybe rode over to Ella's, did something, day in day out, there was no substance. I had to meet with my social worker once a week and she would see me off each time with a "Chinese blessing." How much more wrong could my life get? These social workers didn't understand a word of what I said. They were former drug addicts themselves, you could tell by looking at them and hear it in their eighties slang. Of course, they probably weren't, but in attacks of cold hatred that's what I thought. They were no help to me, only the apartment was a help, but I couldn't have that unless I showed up for the meetings with them. The conversations would dribble along, arduous and meaningless, week after week, and achieve nothing, nothing, nothing. I had to get out of there.

Robert is someone else who helped me get out. He pitched in administratively, wherever he could. The debts that kept piling up and multiplying all by themselves were curbed, regular payments were agreed upon, partial monthly payments were made, guarantees were secured, translation contracts were acquired. We managed to get rid of the uncouth, rather untrustworthy lawyer from Spandau that a court had imposed as an adviser and got

Robert approved instead. We met once a week for lunch, a structuring framework that he maintained. I knew I could turn to him to help put out fires.

I handled a couple of events myself, the launch of *Sickster* for one. In relaxed desperation, I fielded questions and came up with partially witty answers from deep down in my depression, and in the process I learned exactly what kind of humour you can develop if you have nothing more to lose. Spotlights, sweat, panic, the dark faces of the audience didn't matter, didn't matter. I gave a couple of other readings, barely tolerating them. I kept on, barely kept on, crisscrossing Germany by train, more and more despondent. None of that was worthwhile, I thought. None of it is worthwhile. Those are the landscapes, and I am here. Those are the vain people, and I am here. The trees are fresh, but dead, the people are there, but gone. What is all this supposed to be.

And me. What am I supposed to be, supposed to do.

65

The question about how society contributed to my falling ill, and the knowledge that I can only keep on asking this question, making it more precise every time, but never find an answer. Again, no one to blame, just the guilt, which I can only pin on myself. Mechanisms of exclusion, class differences, humiliations, the need to cling to something—it does no good to point the finger at others. If only I could believe in some kind of gods I could accuse and blame. But I can't. It is what it is, and my gaze moves on to a dripping döner kebab on a spike, with the deeply browned meat bubbling and the Turkish German street vendor yelling his pushy, "Yes, please" at the passersby, energetically and noisily sharpening his knife and dully staring at the cars driving by. The wet street is hissing at them, and they're hissing right back. Nothing has changed, nothing is like it used to be.

66

We lost the lawsuit we launched to create a legal precedent for the debts, which drove the debts even higher. Later, I wrote a fictionalized account in *3000 Euros*. I slipped a disc in the worst kind of way, probably because I'd spent the last year charging around with a laptop and books hanging in a shoulder bag. Some people also talked about psychosomatic causes, but I don't know about that. In any case, I couldn't move, I couldn't spend time lying down, or sitting, or standing, or walking, and after three months of medication, shots, physiotherapy, and patience, I finally had an operation. Your body has its own alarm system. Unfortunately, mine was activated far too late.

I could hardly speak in the hospital room. The other patients, who proudly showed off their extensive scars, were in such good moods that I felt like someone who had been isolated for being autistic. Ella visited me every day; Aljoscha came by too, caustic but hearty.

I moved again, after a year and a half, and landed in Neukölln, in the first apartment of my own in ages, because the girlfriend of the girlfriend of my ex-girlfriend reported that the apartment across the landing was vacant. Robert signed the guarantee they required and told the superintendent, "Yes, Thomas has been on a rampage—but that's over and done with!"

Even with the operation, the slipped disc had damaged my body. I'd been left with a slight limp. My psyche was as unfurnished as my apartment, in the shadows, skeptically gazing at itself, leery of thoughts that were too agitated or aggressive and wary of the sedation and flaccidity. Whenever I felt happy, I would hold back and even as the happiness poured forth I folded it back up into a tight little packet. Whenever I daydreamed, I ruthlessly shook myself awake. Whenever melancholy slipped over me, I closed my eyes and waited for it to go away. Mustn't be too happy! Mustn't give in to grief. It was life with a handbrake on. Although I could concentrate again, make new plans, and I actually managed to get a book out during this dead end, I was no longer a complete human being, and I never would be one again.

I was getting better, but was staying sick.

2016

1

The decisive part is that which appears on the screen, as Werner Herzog's film *My Best Fiend* tells us. I am not so sure about that anymore. My books are my screen, but they're not much help; life dissipates, I am just barely holding it together. It may be true that I live only in my writing, which is why this text is not only a report on an illness, a self-abnegation with blind spots, but also a sort of negative mini-cultural history, the anti-*Bildungsroman* that *Sickster* was meant to be, and a bitter jest.

But while the problems on the page have been at least partially resolved, those in life haven't even been touched, even when they're brought together, as they are here.

2

I'm sitting in Neukölln. I hate this neighbourhood. The dull faces, emptied by drink, wreck my mood every time I venture out into the street. They have dead eyes and gravity has dragged their mouths into a downward grimace; the alcoholically enhanced popcorn noses, so-called rosacea, are shining red cauliflower lumps with burst arteries inside, and hair that is sparse and broken has been pulled into a thin little ponytail, perhaps meant to recall long-lost lives in Kreuzberg. Depressed and bowed down by life, such

ponytailed creatures stagger through the streets along-
side un-ponytailed ones and seem to hate Neukölln just
as much as I do. You can see it in their stony faces, the
battered shopping bags, the cheap baked goods: nothing
but a completely shattered present, and a future that in
the best of cases means repeating it all to death. Nobody
here has sold their soul, no, their souls got lost, or never
existed in the first place. The migrants live more isolated
lives than they do in Kreuzberg, which adds to the frosty
disparity of the neighbourhood, as do the Spanish and
American artist-tourists who storm the new cafés and bars
and remain strictly among themselves, then disperse out
into the world again. Nobody here has anything to do with
anybody else, and the vibe is either stupidly upscale or dull
and grungy. There's one internet café after another, with
a few shisha bars in between that apparently exist mainly
for money-laundering purposes, and then an inhumane,
futuristically cold shopping mall packed full of strange
shops. And quickly assembled bars with pretentious patch-
work people inside, full of themselves and yet oh so empty.

3

Life has left its mark. This truism is particularly apt in my
case. The average but nevertheless still-present attractive-
ness that people attributed to me in my twenties has been
lost in the increasing lumpiness of my appearance. Medications have played their role. They're meant to save me
but at the same time they work against me. I have bloated
over the past years, long weighing over a hundred kilos.
The rather agile body of the young man I once was has,
over years of medication and paralyzing excess, been rendered clumsy and heavy. Week by week this grows more
disturbing: the result is Tarantino with a shot of Jabba the

Hutt. And the acne keeps on taking over parts of my face. I've spent too much time sleeping and I've slept too heavily, without the pleasure of a single dream. But I've had to sleep, as much as possible, to ward off any danger. My libido dropped almost to zero. Uninterested, I would observe the opposite sex the way a middle-class citizen observes a work of art, with pleasure but without any lust or greed. If I did feel any impulse, I would usually just ignore it. And I lived my ambitionless life with the same lack of interest, yes, the same uninterested displeasure, experiencing it as a series of mandatory events I would usually try to avoid. Even without the medication and the therapy, this could well be my condition, but the suspicion that those chemical bombardments have damaged my body and my mind and taken them hostage does not go away. And the daily ransom money I receive in small change is called normality.

The illness ages you decades before your time, both physically and mentally: it accelerates the wear and tear. At the same time, a core of immaturity glimmers on within you, a part that fights off any development and remains inert. That is the relic of the times before madness set in and medication triumphed, a sealed off leftover "I" that cannot be expunged. It yearns for the old life and, independent of my will, clings to it and to itself. And so you grow old, but you don't grow up.

4

My illness deprived me of my home. Now my illness is my home. But things are getting better, always better. I've been able to breathe freely for two years now. Not everything is illness. It's possible to have a normal conversation with me again. Soon I will have paid off the last remaining debts. At some point I will have to organize my accounts and finish things up. Then it'll be time for a new apartment, the last one for a long time I hope, and finally, who knows, the novel that will cover the entire spectrum of society. That hasn't been possible so far, because my damn life kept pushing its way into my writing, the illness forcing its way in. I did not choose this topic for my life.

A year and a half, two years, two and a half years: altogether six years. Bipolar disorder stole six years of my life. So I am really thirty-five years old but physically I'm fifty-three, and on the inside I alternate between being seven and seventy.

5

The shadow cannot be easily erased. While others might be diagnosed with a depressive mood disorder, in my case, with all the conditions and contortions, it can be said to be a constant state of mind. Others would go to the hospital, I go to the movies. I'm satisfied with little and just want to carry on. And I'm even thinking about maybe doing some sports.

Self-flagellation, after all, is just a counter-clockwise twist on vanity. And paranoia a particularly morbid form of narcissism. An end to all that.

But I'm afraid that in this decade of isolation I may have lost touch with the manners and cultural techniques I spent years working to acquire and may end up living my life as a weirdo outsider, subject to thousands of tics, from pulling out my hair to holding my breath. I'm afraid of losing more of what is inside me, the way I lost my books. I am struck with disproportionate sorrow when my old telephone numbers come to mind but I can't remember my current one. When I do want to recall it, I just remember fragments of the old ones. That gets me down and shows me where my head is at.

My head still dreams about them, I mean, it's still dreaming about my books in long futuristic dreams, in fantasies of reconciliation during endless special U-Bahn journeys that take me to book fairs where I participate as a browser, not an invited author, and I pack my enormous bags full to the brim with precious, gorgeous, freshly printed books that I carefully pre-selected at home. And at the book fair I meet up with everybody, and they've all forgiven me long ago, and I show them the books that we'll enjoy together.

6

Then there's this Beckett moment when I wake up from dozing in total nothingness, and pure panic takes hold, frightened scrabbling to get up, senseless feverishness that translates into jerky movements and can be assuaged only with cigarettes. But that is my existence. There is nothing more. That's it. That's you, naked, in Being-ness, nothing but muscles and shaky handwriting. The perspective of an alien or an animal or just the *world*, that you need to briefly take in and immediately abandon, in horror: the human-free observation of humans. Two eyes, nerves, signals resonating.

The same perspective took hold of me during my most recent readings. I had panic attacks that put all other previous panic attacks in the shade. I was suddenly struck silent. I couldn't utter a word, I was hyperventilating. The audience sat there, helpless and staring. A woman produced a package of glucose candy. A journalist later wrote that my "verbal functions" had evidently dropped to "absolutely nil." This may come from the blurring of fiction and autobiography, from the fact that I was never able to be completely honest about my earlier work, which always veiled the relationship between the protagonists and the author. Maybe my attempt in this book to establish the two identities as distinct will help. But maybe I just can't do it.

How is it that a working-class kid from a dysfunctional background, intellectually pimped up by the Jesuits, sent out into the literary world by Nabokov, and theory-infected by the nothing-counts-anymore postmodernism at university, all this mixed up with genetic factors, is supposed to turn himself into a poet? Or even a happy person? Give me a break!

My greatest comfort: medical experience has shown that a temporarily complete recovery from this disease is always possible, is even the rule—you just don't know if it will last for months, or for years, or forever. The psychotic and paranoid elements do not become chronic. The madness is almost always a temporary phenomenon and rarely ends in permanent derangement or dementia. The illness is only chronic in that it always returns. It is a threat. That threatens, and threatens, and threatens.

When I read the medical texts and the prognoses, I sometimes feel like simply taking my leave. The rate of relapse is so high, despite medication, and so scary, that I feel like just lying down to sleep forever. Reading these pages makes my heart race, and then stall in sadness.

There is a promise in pop music, in poetry, in film, that life simply cannot fulfill. I remain wrapped up in this promise and observe life only from outside. Arno Schmidt: "The life of art and fantasy is the only reality, the rest is a nightmare."

Better get back to fiction, and soon. It'll work out, it will. The images are sliding into each other, gradually becoming one.

7

Hamburg, Schulterblatt Strasse: I have to look up the places I scorched in my mania, have to banish and neutralize them. Saal II, for instance, and a waiter by the name of Hagen. But other bars, pubs, and restaurants too, that I walk past, that I stop at. One glance and the curse is lifted, at least for a few days. It's not so easy with people.

8

Back in Neukölln, I observe the showdown of the endbosses. A turf war between two crazy tramps from the neighbourhood culminates before my eyes in a huge screaming fit. One of them, who has the look of a dead young boy on her old-woman face, has been roaming around the block for a while, for the last year or two. She'll growl at you, mutter to herself, and then spout incomprehensible invective; it's hard to figure out. She usually spends the day doing crossword puzzles on the sill of the basement window where she also spends the night. The other woman, somewhat younger, more wiry and energetic, but also acutely crazier and palpably more dangerous, has been in the hood for about two weeks. She has already come on to me, she clearly hates herself, hates the people and the neighbourhood. I am present the day the two of them meet up, recognize each other as competitors, and start screaming. The local tramp soon wanders off, apparently conceding defeat, while the new arrival, armed with a stick, keeps after her, yelling. Then she loses track. A day later, I see the new woman again, the stick has become her companion, she's screaming out orders at the intersection. Then she disappears, and the tramp with the older claim moves back onto her basement windowsill as though nothing happened. Stuck between empathy and disgust, I have grown impassive—like the others—in the face of this misery. I am one of them. And I am one of the others.

9

Back at home, the machines kicked into action again, like every morning, old, unmodern things that set to work clattering and hissing to pump coffee or gas through the pipes and holes with me at the receiving end, sitting there all alone again and consuming whatever it was they produced: the hot water tank, the flow heater, the coffee machine, out of date and with encrustations and, all in all, sinfully expensive. I stood there in the apartment, motionless, it was still morning, listening to the creaks and whispers that came from the heating system and the thermostat. There was a smell of nicotine, sleep, and farewell.

10

Oh I do believe
In all the things you see
What comes is better than what came
Before

11

My book collection is forever lost, but slowly, very slowly, there is another one growing at my back. Other people choose to sell off their books and see that as progress, with Kindles in hand and three months' reading paid for at an optimized flat rate. I was an old-fashioned fellow, a guy who despite all my affinity for the internet had a different, older concept of literature, with a book collection at my back and alcohol on my breath. I failed as a traditionalist. This fossil is no more. Everything can start anew. Freedom is burgeoning as a result.

The world at my back, I will not give up. My hope is never to go manic again. But it may knock me down and carry me away once more, then have me wash up as some boneless jellyfish. I will just have to earn back my bones with hard work. If I do succumb to another mania, I hope someone will hand me this book. If I do go mad again, I will accept that as my fate. After my second bout, I thought I would not survive a third one. But I did. And I would again. I may want to kill myself again, at some point. Then I will live on still.

Then these lines will be like a prayer.

Born in Bonn, Germany, THOMAS MELLE studied at the University of Tübingen, the University of Texas at Austin, and the Free University of Berlin. His novels *Sickster* and *3000 Euros* were finalists for the German Book Prize in 2011 and 2014 respectively. Melle is also a prolific playwright and translator. His translations from English to German have ranged from plays by William Shakespeare to novels by William T. Vollmann. *The World at My Back*, also a finalist for the German Book Prize, was a bestseller in Germany. It was made into a highly successful stage play, and has been translated into eighteen languages.

Thomas Melle lives in Berlin.

LUISE VON FLOTOW teaches translation studies at the University of Ottawa School of Translation and Interpretation. Her recent translations include, from German, *They Divided the Sky* by Christa Wolf, and *Everyone Talks About the Weather...We Don't* by Ulrike Meinhof; and, from French, *The Four Roads Hotel* by France Théoret. She has twice been a finalist for the Governor General's Award for Literary Translation.

Biblioasis International Translation Series
General Editor: Stephen Henighan